# DRUG CALCULATIONS FOR NURSES WHO HATE

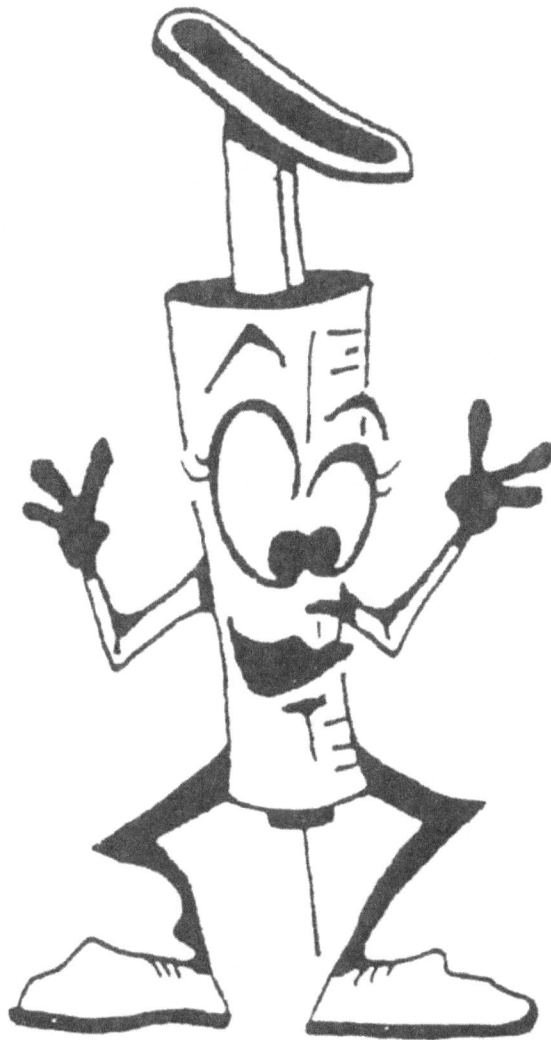

# NUMBERS

By: Malcolm Rosenberg RN

*Illustrated by: Scott Brown*

# DRUG CALCULATIONS
# FOR
# NURSES WHO HATE NUMBERS

## MALCOLM ROSENBERG, R.N.

### Illustrated by Scott Brown

Malcom Rosenberg
370 N.W. 115 Way
Coral Springs, FL 3071
(954) 753-5915

Copyrighted 1992
Printed in the United States of America

To
Craig, Alex and Sandy
for three diffrent kinds of love
and
Iris Perez without whom I could not
have written this book.

# INTRODUCTION

I am someone for whom many things did not come easily. Many times, after having learned something, I could not believe how easy it could have been - things that I had struggled with for years.

During my long stay in nursing school (a good example of unnecessary difficulty), I have seen many students struggle with the mathematics of drug calculations. As someone who had previously struggled with numbers (another example) I have been quite successful in explaining this material to students who hate numbers.

As I drew pitcures, did examples, made analogies and anything else to explain the material this book wrote itself. I believe that the same pictures, examples and analogies that worked for my fellow students will work for you.

I know that you can learn the material from this book. I also want you to enjoy the task - which is why I wrote this book.

Malcolm Rosenberg

Since you all don't especially like numbers, I have reduced the units you must learn to four kinds.

Now because I have not included minims, drams, Roman Numerals, centigrams and hectoliters please learn what little I ask. Then we'll both succeed. In other words, I'm depending on you to make me look good.

The units are Liter, Milliliter, Gram and Milligram. If you know these, the rest you can look up later. Let's look at what they are.

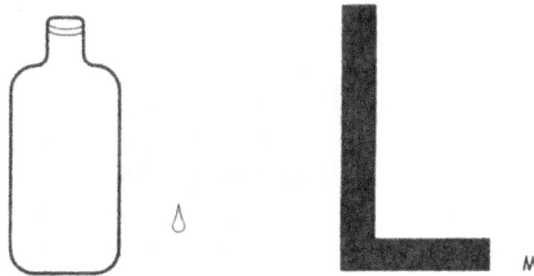

## LITER TO MILLILITER RATIO

A **Liter** is almost the same as a quart (5.5 % larger to be exact.) There are 1000 **Milliliters** in a liter. For the purposes of this chapter, and later chapters, I would recommend getting a small syringe and squirting exactly one calibrated Milliliter. Try squirting a friend. It will break up the monotony of drug mathematics.

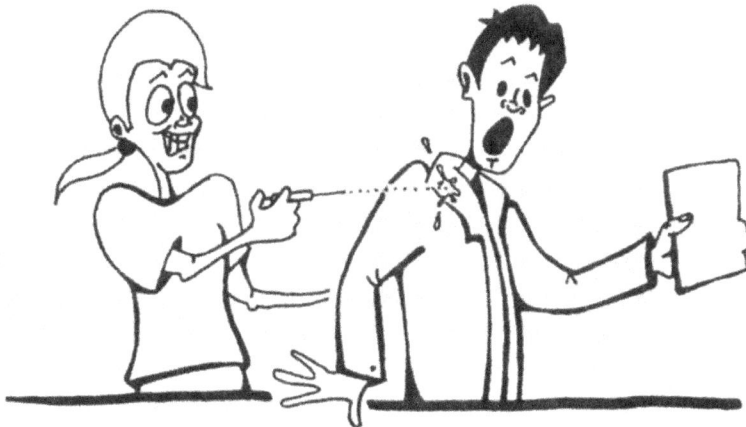

Next is **Grams**. This paper clip weighs 1/2 gram. So two paper clips weigh 1 gram.

Next is **Milligram**. 1000 milligrams equals one gram - that's not very heavy. I can't think of anything that weighs a milligram. A pin weights about 50mg.

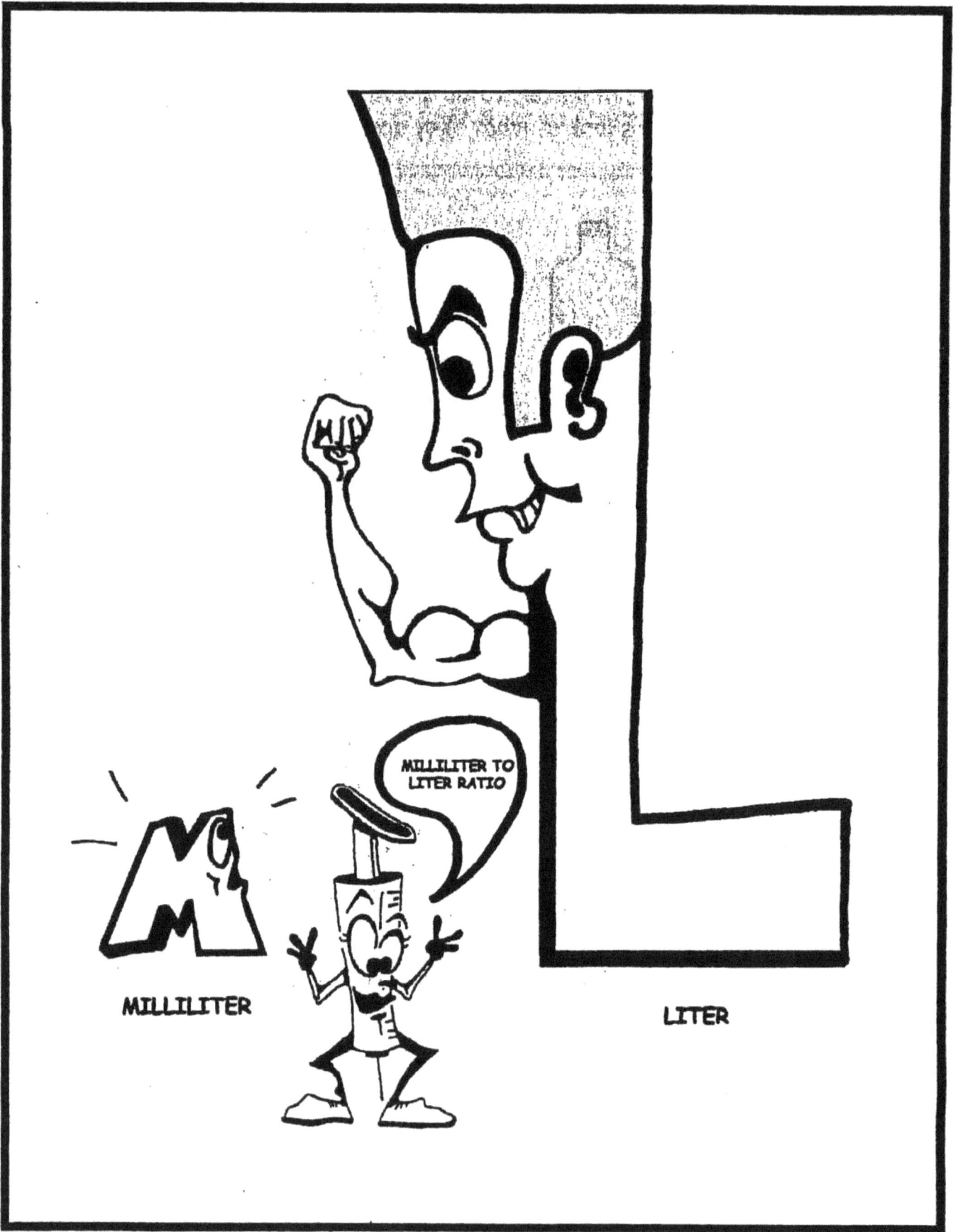

MILLILITER TO LITER RATIO

MILLILITER

LITER

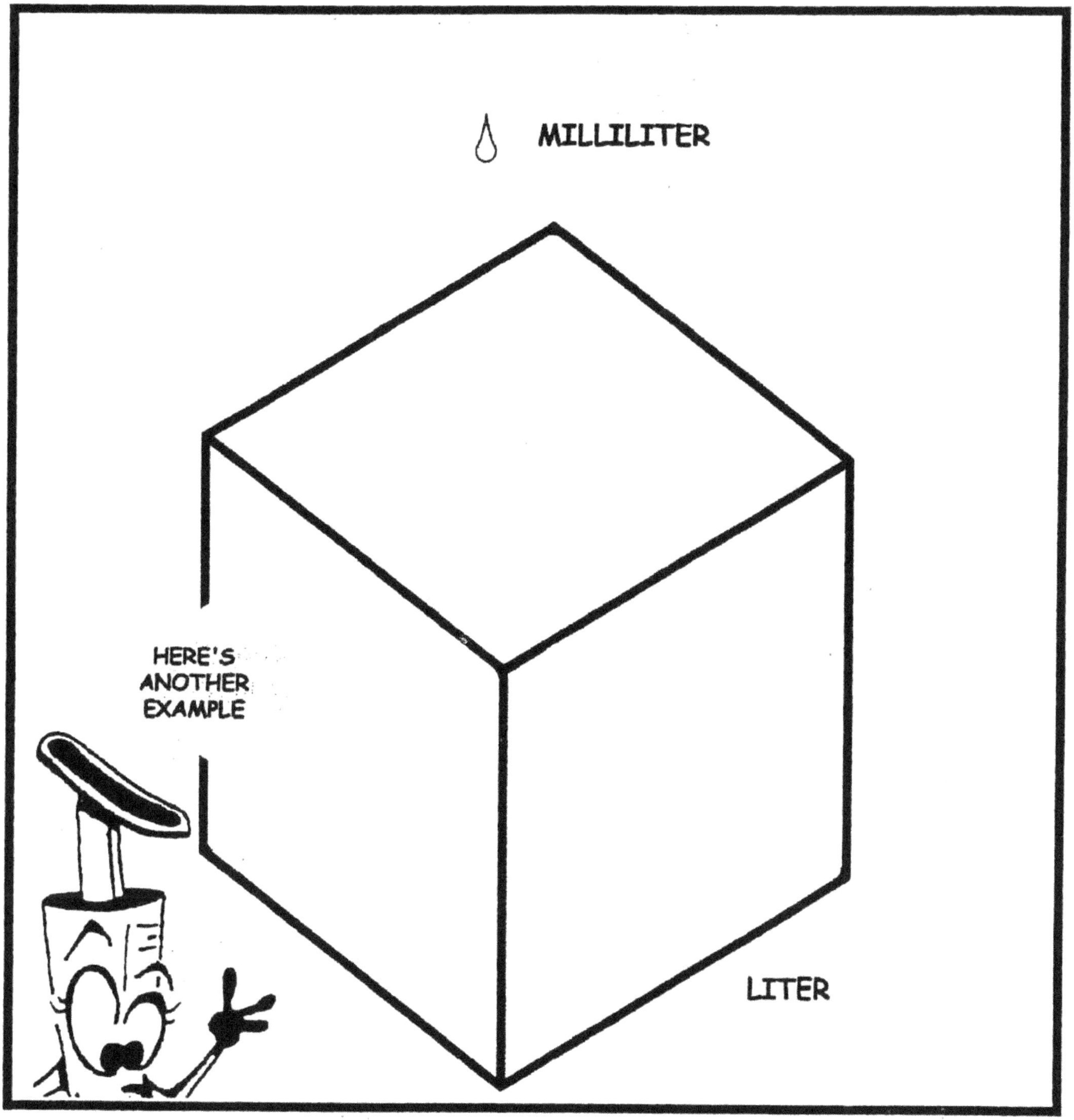
MILLILITER
HERE'S ANOTHER EXAMPLE
LITER

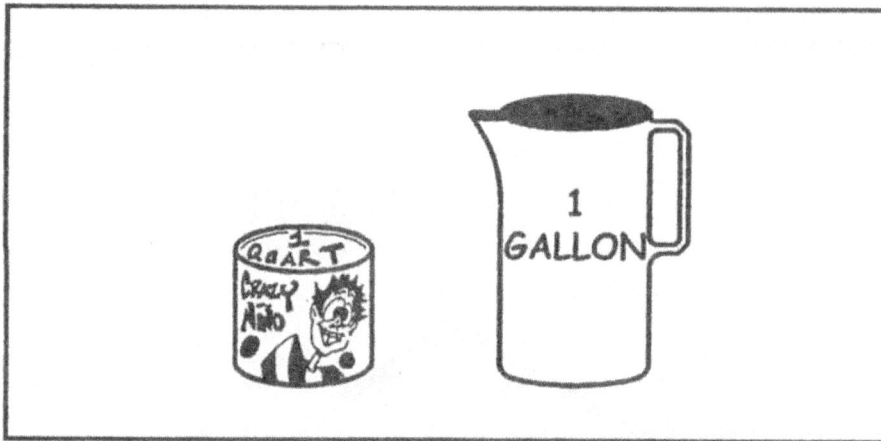

I'm going to make an important point. So pay attention. I'll always try to wake everybody up when we're coming to a good part.

The word is **Active Ingredient**. Lets look at a Coca-Cola from McDonalds. They take about 5ml of syrup, add a pint of water and a little fizz and charge 89 cents. Why do they dilute the Real Thing?

> 1.) you'd get it in a shot glass
> 2.) they couldn't charge 89 cents
> 3.) it would be awfully potent

So what we'll be learning is how much syrup you'd put in a smaller or larger Coca-Cola and still taste just as refreshing.

What was the point of that minor diversion from medication? The point is that we are doing exactly the same thing with a $62.00 life saving antibiotic as a refreshing Coca-Cola.

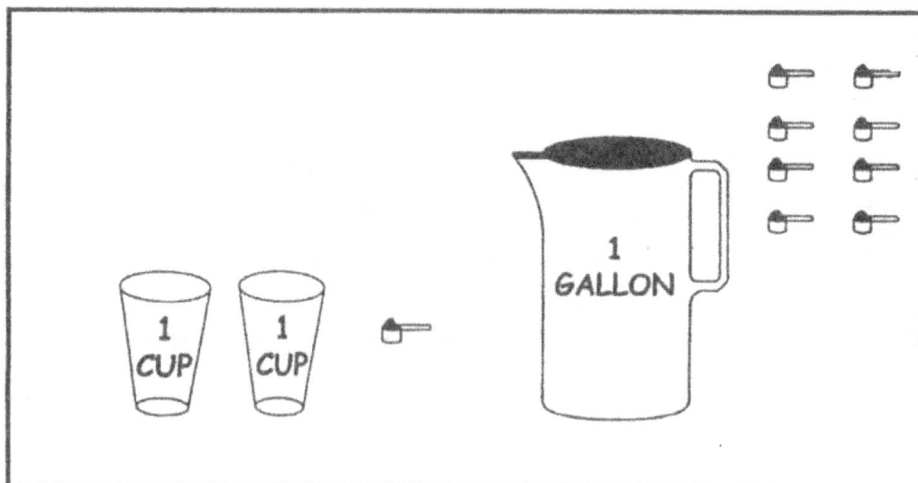

Now for some hands on experience with ratio and proportion, we'll use Kool-Aid. According to the directions on the package one scoop of powder added to 2 large glasses serves 2 people. For that same delicious taste, it tells us to add two scoops to a quart and adding 8 scoops to a gallon is definitely a party.

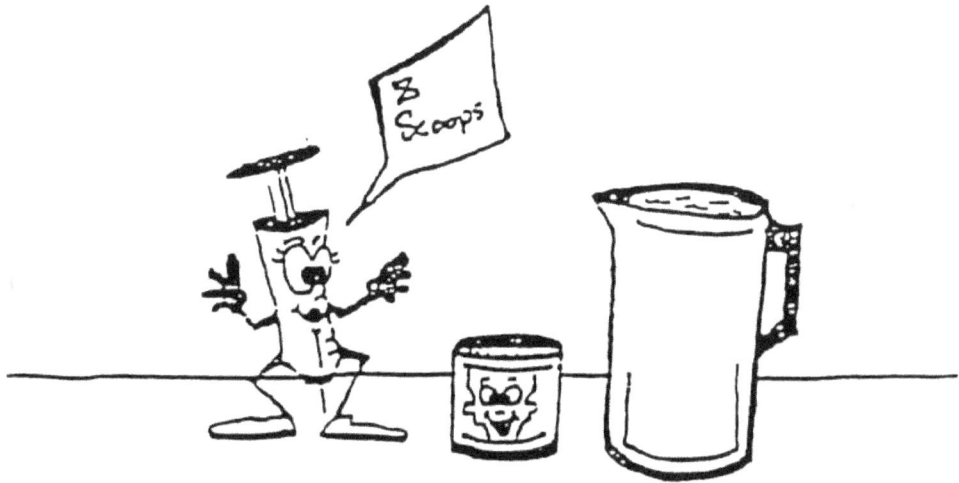

Anyway, it's the active ingredient (the powder, not the water) we are concerned with because that's what gives Kool Aid its kick, not too much and not too little.  Too little and it would taste like dishwater.  Too much and it would be too sweet.

How many scoops would we put in one glass?  The directions told us one scoop, for two large glasses.

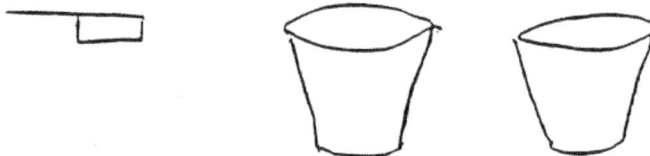

So for one large glass, how many scoops do we want?  Half as much drink in one glass.  Half as much powder for one glass.  One half scoop of Kool Aid powder for one glass.

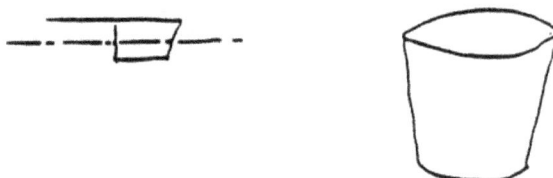

How much water would we need to add?  Well....the amount of drink we're going to want to drink is 1/2, so the amount of water we'll add is also 1/2, one glass.  Let's try a few more.

The instructions say two scoops for a quart.  How many scoops would you add to a gallon of water?

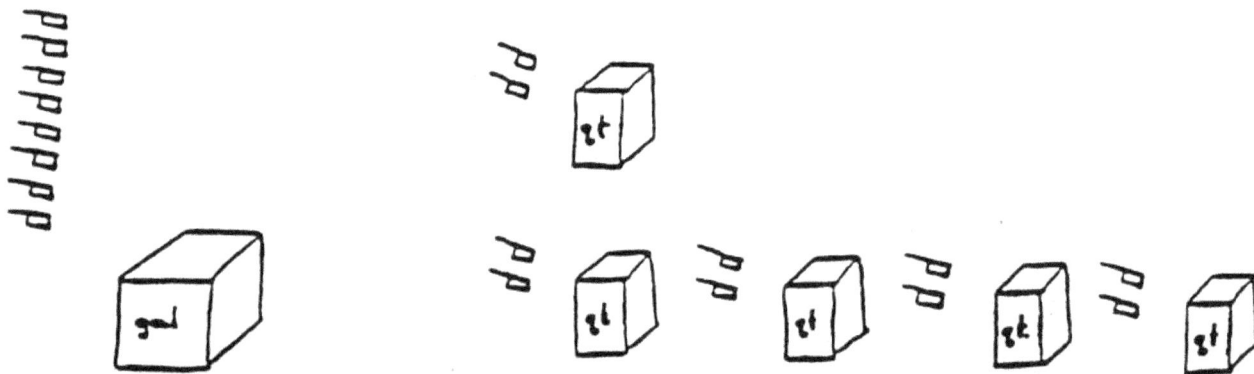

There is 4 times as much water to add to, so we'll add 4 times as much powder.

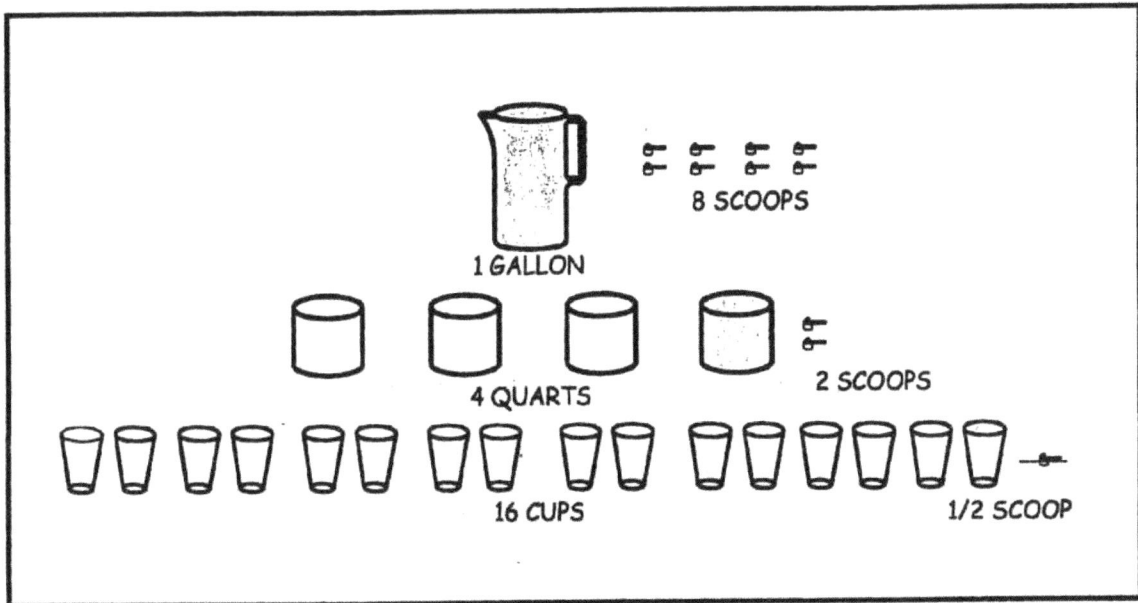

1 GALLON

8 SCOOPS

4 QUARTS

2 SCOOPS

16 CUPS

1/2 SCOOP

This may be getting tedious. But please bear with me, it does progress to medications and exactly what you need to know.

Let's try working the other way. Suppose you were given a gallon of mixed Kool Aid. You poured yourself a cup and your mother said, "That stuff is all sugar, how much of that powder do you put in each cup?" To answer her intelligently we would work backward - and not just look on the last page. We could do this in two steps. First we work back to quarts in a gallon. So a quart would take 1/4 as much powder. 1/4 of 8 scoops is 2 scoops. And further we know there are four large cups in a quart so we would need 1/4 as much powder or 1/4 of two scoops is 1/2 a scoop. That's the answer -1/2 scoop per cup.

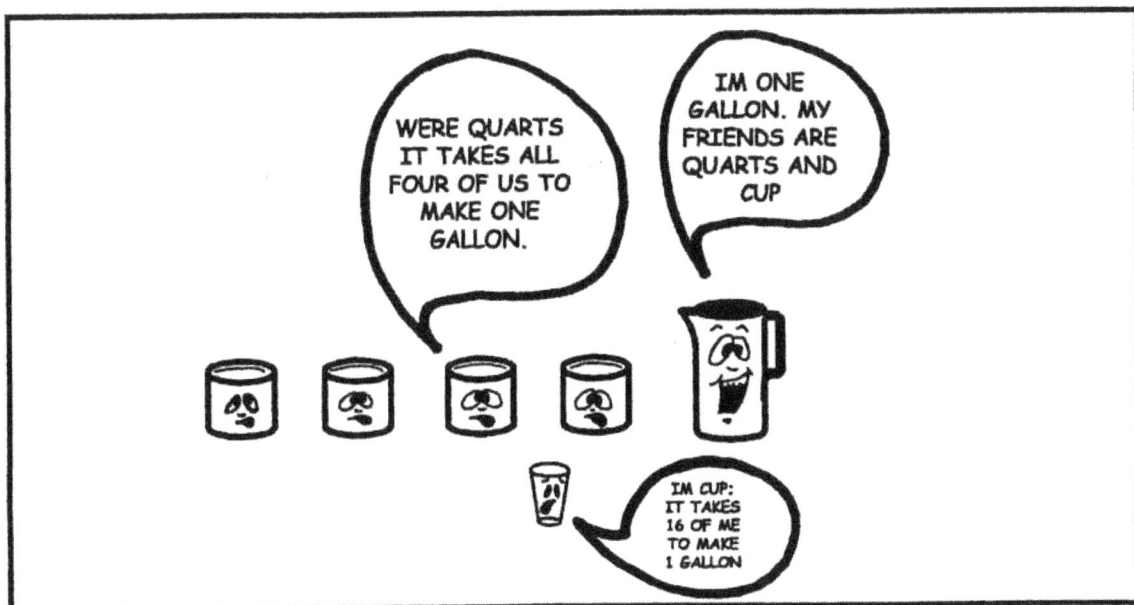

WERE QUARTS IT TAKES ALL FOUR OF US TO MAKE ONE GALLON.

IM ONE GALLON. MY FRIENDS ARE QUARTS AND CUP

IM CUP: IT TAKES 16 OF ME TO MAKE 1 GALLON

I want to do one more of those. Suppose we were at a picnic with a 5 gallon cooler of Kool Aid and all you knew is that you had added 40 scoops of Kool Aid, and someone asked you how much Kool Aid was in his glass. Let's look at this problem in pitcures. We'll work backwards the same way. First to gallons.

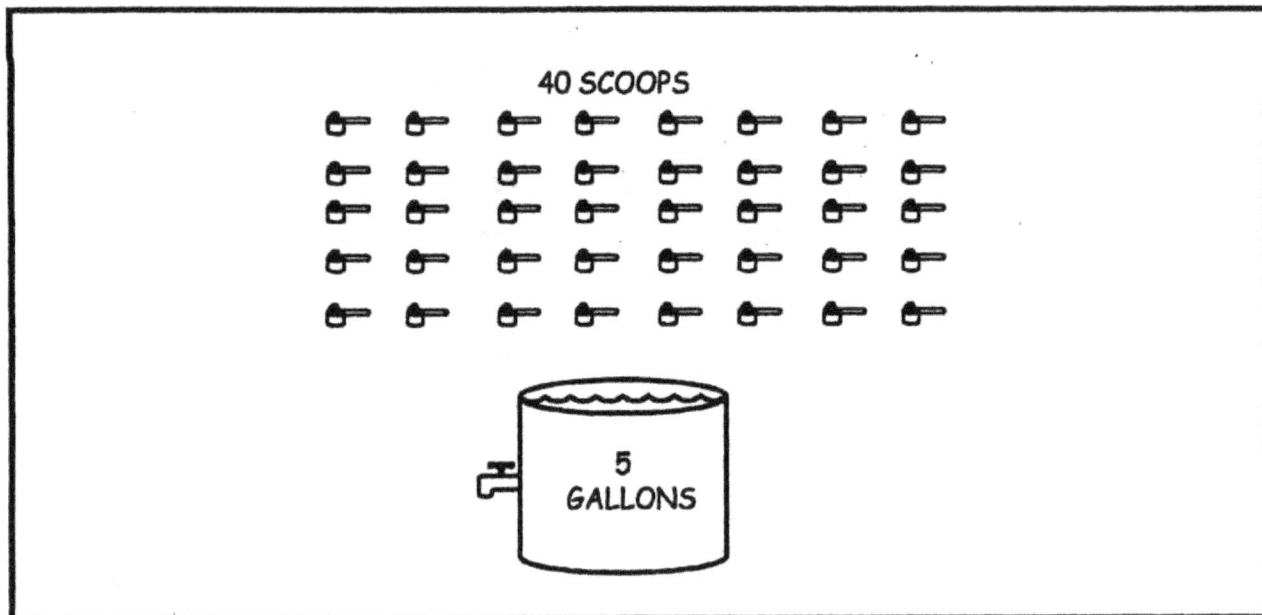

40 SCOOPS

5 GALLONS

Each gallon is 1/5 of the total Kool Aid so the powder is 1/5 of all the powder added. We divide 5 gallons by five to get one gallon and we divide 40 scoops by five to get the powder in each gallon.

$$\frac{5 \text{ GALLONS}}{5} = \frac{40 \text{ SCOOPS}}{5} = 1 \text{ GALLON} = 8 \text{ SCOOPS}$$

Do you see how dividing 5 gallons of Kool Aid and dividing 40 scoops of powder by the same number will give us the scoops of powder in the new amount of Kool Aid? It turns out to be the answer we already know. One gallon of Kool Aid would need 8 scoops.

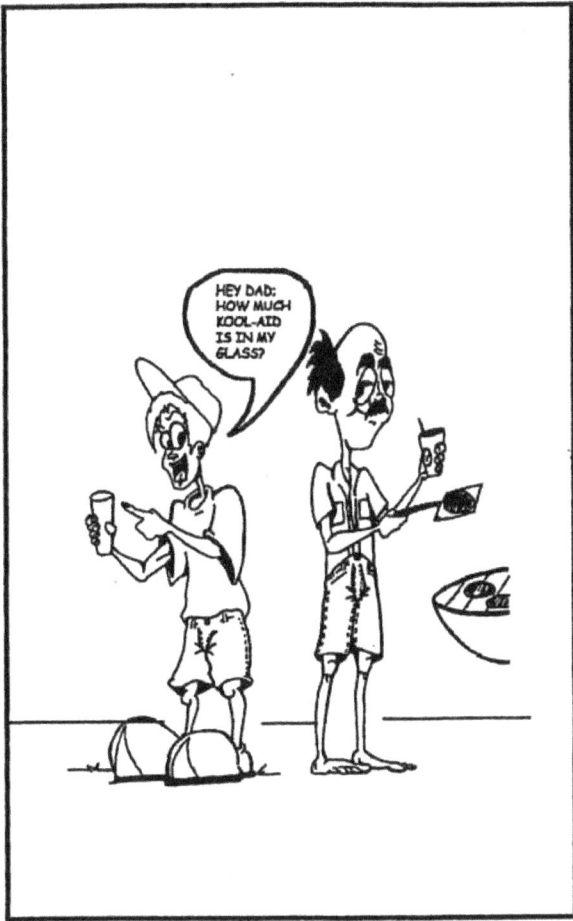

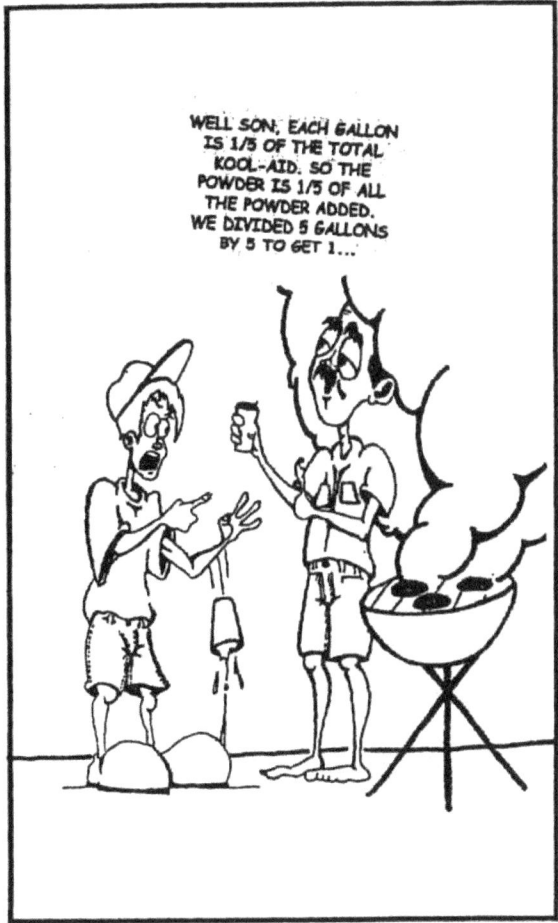

# ISN'T THIS FUN!

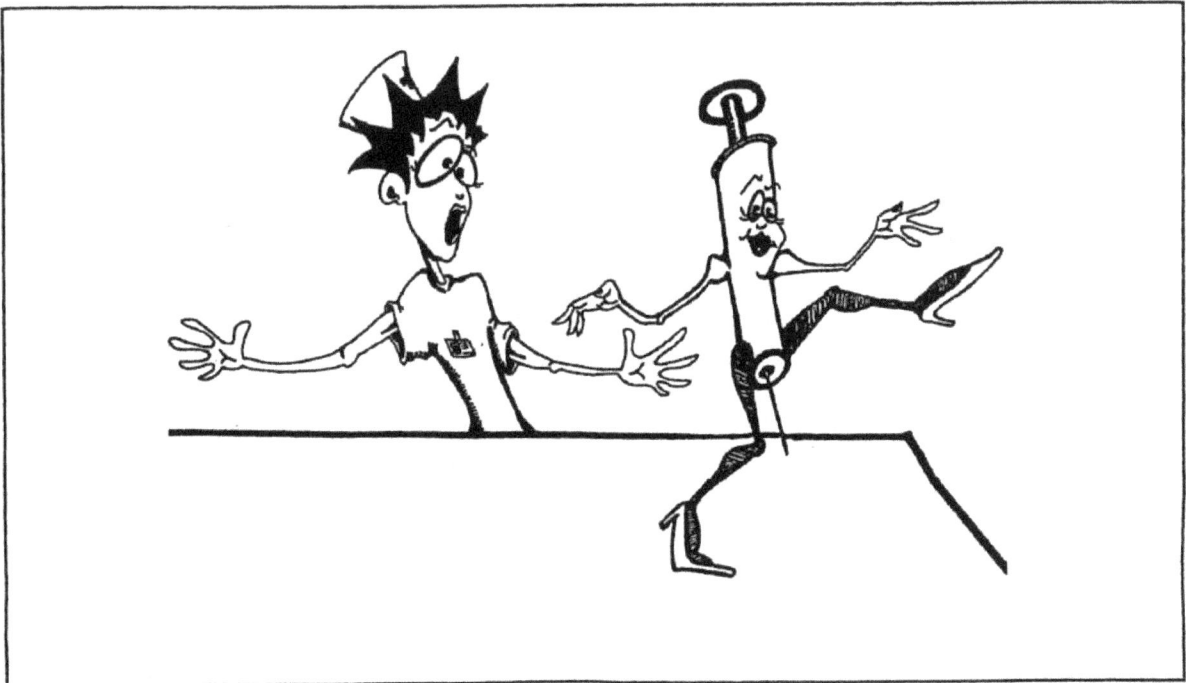

Now working back to quarts, we just calculated 8 scoops of Kool Aid to a gallon. How many scoops in a quart? We know there are 4 quarts in a gallon. Let's take a look at the same picture of scoops and quarts.

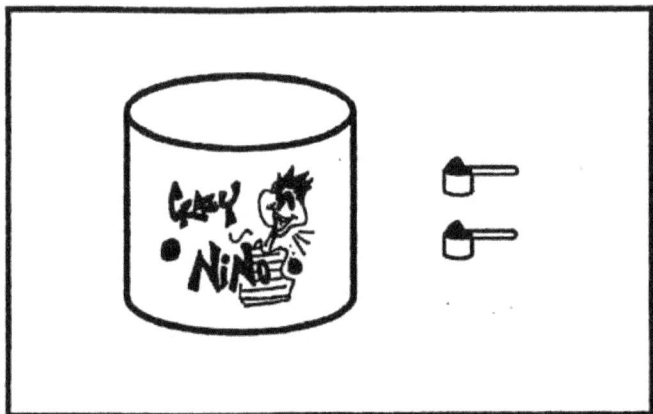

Dividing both gallons and scoops in a gallon by four gives us the number of scoops in one quart or:

1 quart= 4 quarts/4            8 scoops per gallon=
                    2 scoops per quart

And each quart has 2 scoops. Now lets continue working down to glasses. We know one quart is 4 glasses and one quart has 2 scoops. How many scoops in each glass?

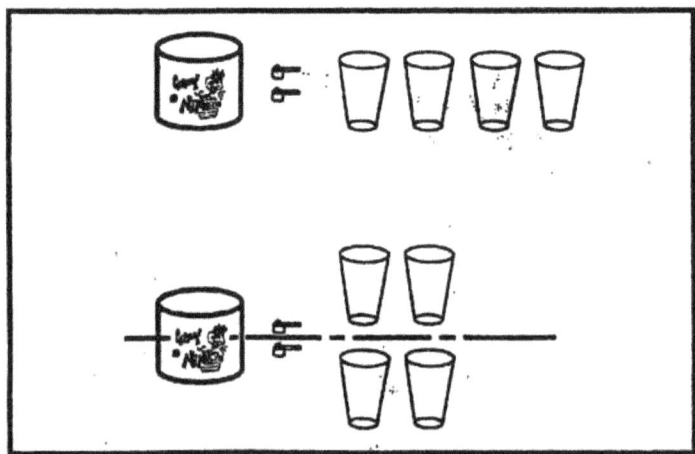

By dividing both the number of glasses and number of scoops in one quart by the same number, we get the number of scoops in each glass.
If you knew that there were 80 glasses in that 5 gallon cooler you could have divided the 40 scoops by 80 glasses to get 1/2 scoop per glass.

Let's try to keep this discussion moving in the right direction. Suppose somebody got a small burst of energy from the sugar. That's not unreasonable. Certainly Snickers would have us believe that. And you knew how much sugar it took to get you going. By these methods you could calculate how much Kool Aid you would have to drink for that little kick. In the previous example your mother was right. Kool Aid is mostly sugar with a little flavoring.

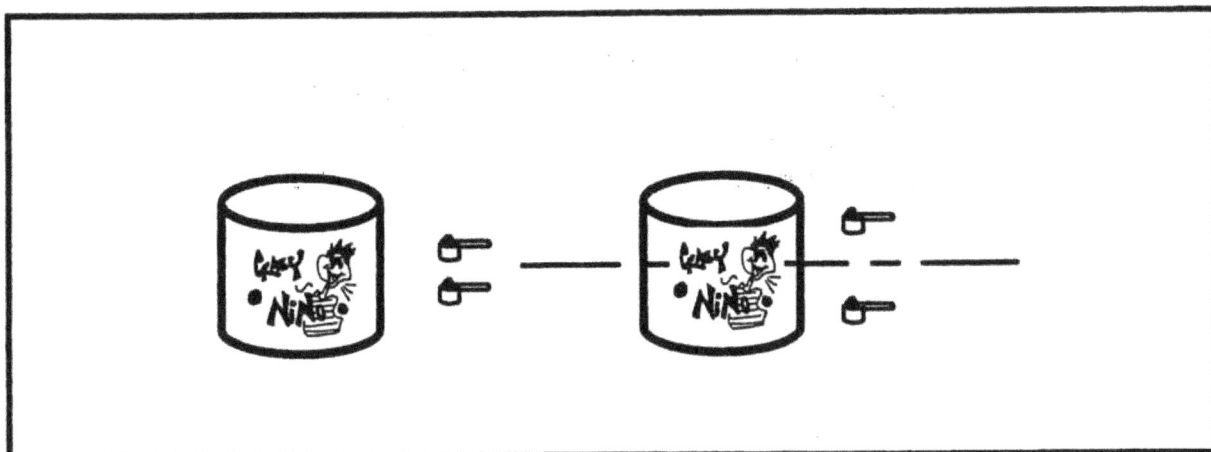

What if one scoop of sugar (Kool Aid) gave you that late afternoon burst of energy? How much water would you add?

If 1/2 scoop mixes with one glass, one scoop would mix with two glasses. To say that another way: suppose we had already mixed a quart couldn't you just pour two glasses for your scoop of sugar?

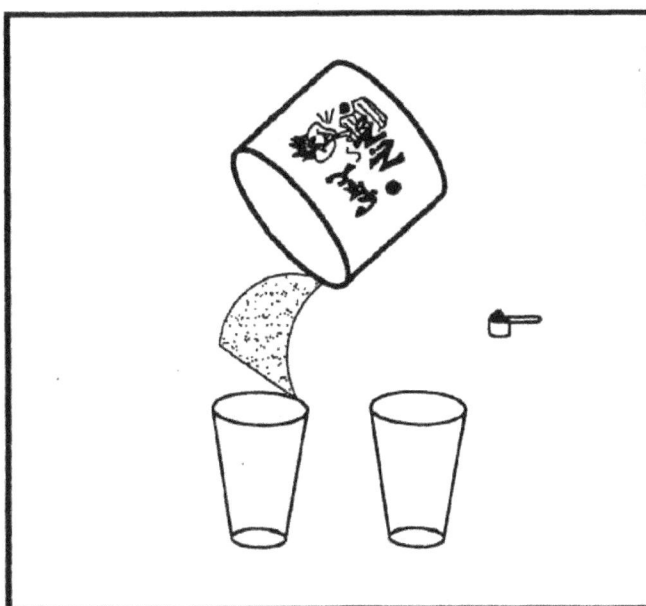

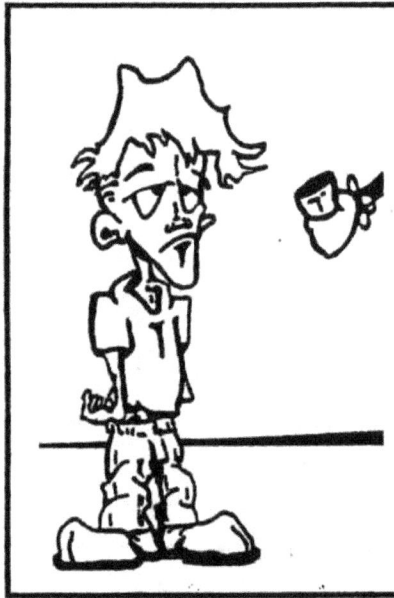

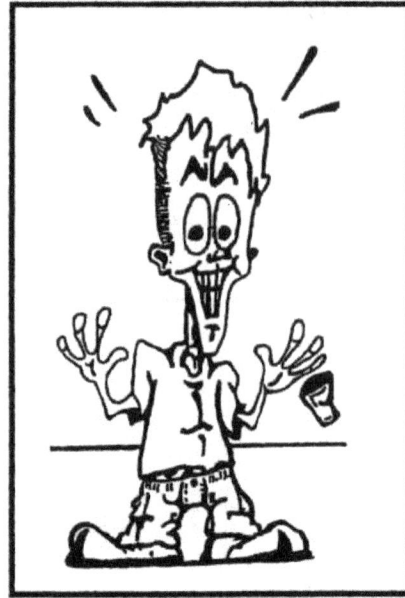

Let's try a few examples with our quart that's already mixed.

Suppose we wanted 1 1/2 scoops, how much Kool aid would be poured? You get two scoops from the whole quart, and get one scoop from a half-quart.

It would be more than 1/2 quart and less than a full quart. How much? Now we are right on the heart of the matter. Lets look at a picture showing the quart and the amount mixed with it————————————

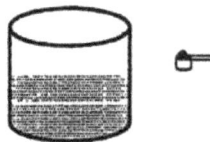

We want all of one scoop. So we would want all of the lower 1/2 quart and half of the upper scoop. So we would also want half the upper half-quart. And that's the answer: 1/2 + 1/4 = 3/4 quart.

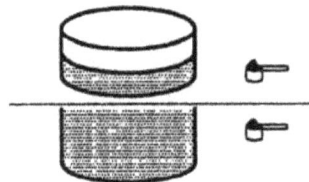

Want to go on to drugs?

# Let's look at something more medicinal

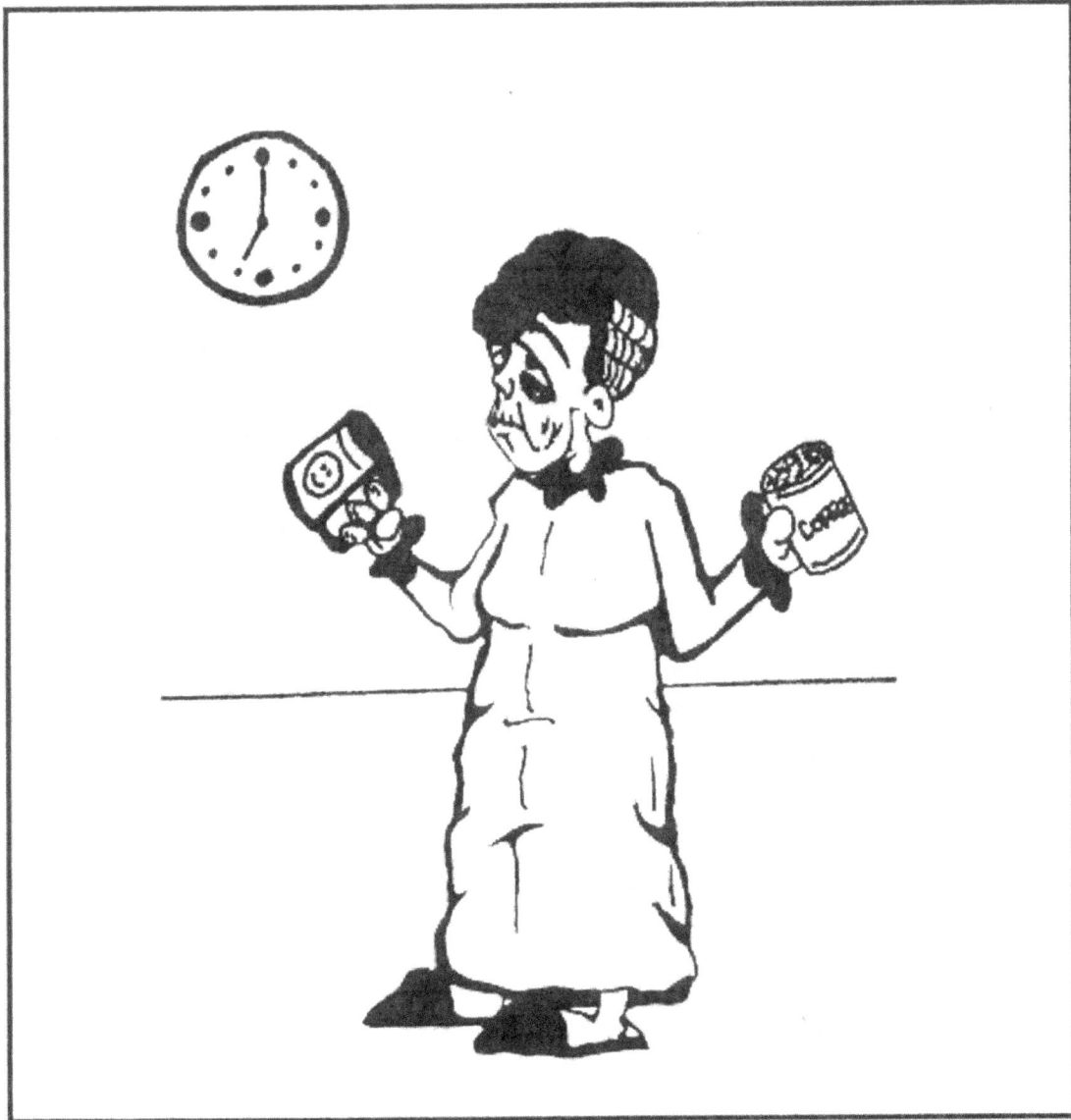

like coffee...

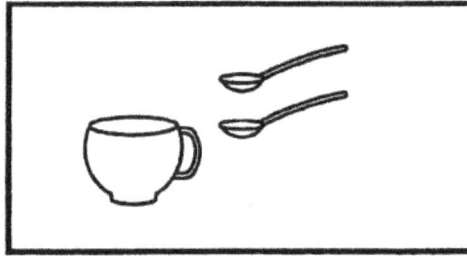

Suppose you added two teaspoons of instant coffee to a cup. And you know from experience that it took one teaspoon to wake you up. How much coffee would you have to drink for your morning fix?

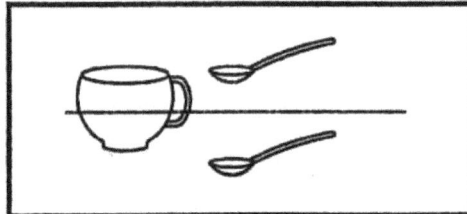

From the picture it should be obvious that half a cup would contain one teaspoon of instant coffee. What if you had built up a tolerance to caffeine and needed 1 1/2 teaspoons? We have already determined that you have to drink the first half cup for one teaspoon .

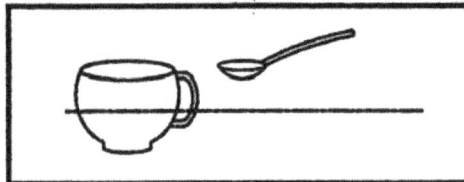

How about the next half teaspoon?

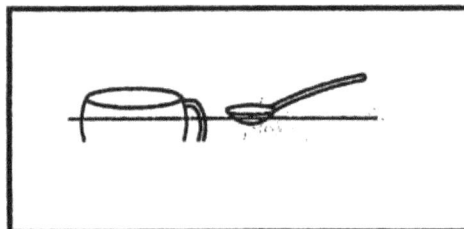

To get 1 1/2 teaspoons we would need half of the top half.

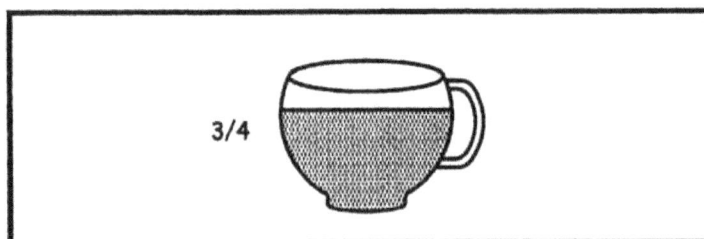

So we would need the bottom half-and-half of the top half to give us 1 1/2 teaspoons. That adds up to three-quarters.

# I COULDN'T HAVE SAID IT BETTER MYSELF....

**Oxydose™**
(oxycodone hydrochloride)
Oral CONCENTRATE Solution  CII

**20 mg/1 mL**

NDC 581-77-914-01

**Dropper Enclosed**
1 fl oz (30 mL)

## PHARMACIST/NURSE/ PATIENT:

**Administration with Dropper:**
Please note the diagram to the right. Fill the dropper to the level of the prescribed dose. For ease of administration, add the dose to approximately 30 mL (1 fl oz) or more of juice or other liquid. May also be added to applesauce, pudding or other semi-solid foods. The drug-food mixture should be used immediately and not stored for future use.

Return dropper to bottle after use.

**Discard Opened Bottle After 90 Days.**

Protect From Light

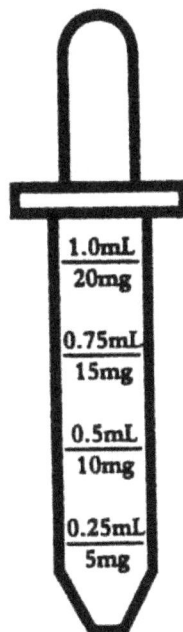

1.0mL
20mg

0.75mL
15mg

0.5mL
10mg

0.25mL
5mg

**Oxydose™**
(oxycodone hydrochloride)
Oral CONCENTRATE Solution  CII

# SUMMARY

What we've been doing is finding the smallest useful unit of active ingredients, scoops of Kool Aid or teaspoons of coffee.

The reason is that it is useful to find out how much active ingredient is in the smallest unit. Then you can work up and down the scale. Let's try one more example before we go on to drugs. Suppose oranges were $1.20 a dozen, and you wanted three. It would be easy to figure the cost of three oranges, if you knew they were 10c each. That would be much easier than figuring that 3 is 1/4of a dozen and 1/4 of $1.20 is 30c.

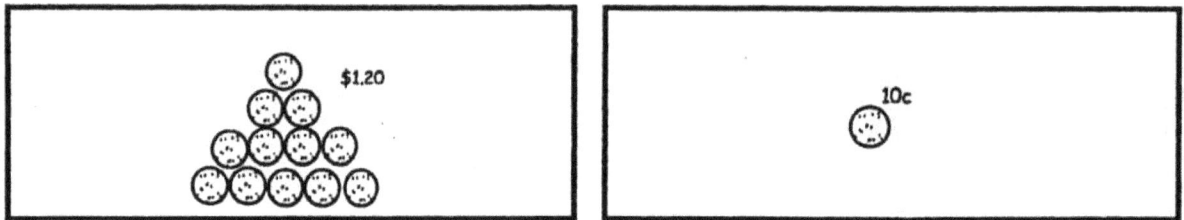

## DRUGS......at last

Versed is often given before gastrointestinal procedures. It comes in 5ml vial. The concentration is one mg to ml

The active 5mg ingredient is totally diluted in 5ml. But for our purposes we'll show 5 individual milligrams in 5 individual milliliters.

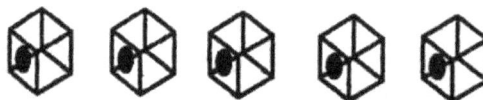

What we want to do first is determine the smallest unit of **active ingredients** that we need. Then we refer to the problem to see how many we are asked to give and finally determine the **volume** or **milliliters** that we need to dispense.

In this case milligrams and milliliters are the units we'll use. What if the doctor orders 3mg? That's three milliliters - which is the volume we would draw from the ampule and inject.

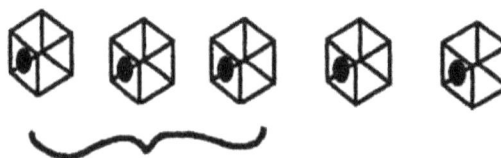

Let's look at most popular drug there is ...aspirin. Aspirin as you get it on the shelf is 325mg... that is 325mg of acetal salielic acid **"Active Ingredient"** the aspirin pill weighs about 1 gram.

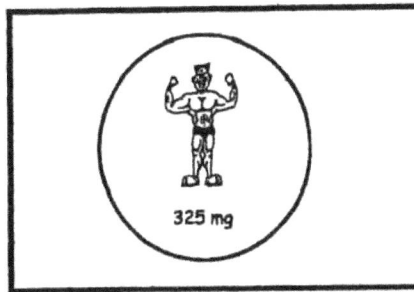

Most people take two aspirin at a time. How much active ingredient are they getting in two tablets.

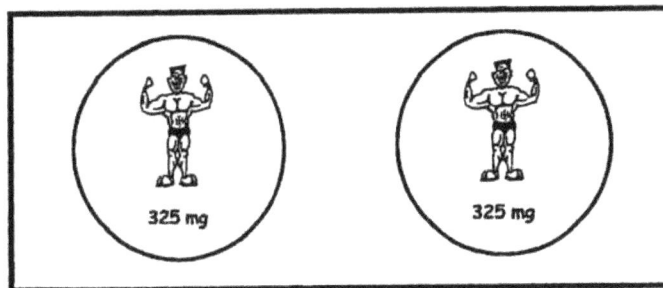

Another 325mg analgesic tablet is acetaminophen. Two tablets would give you 650mg of active ingredient.

A stonger version comes in 500mg tablets 500mg of active ingredient even though the pill is the same size.

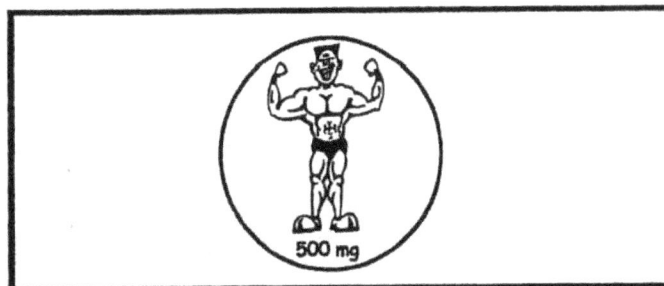

One pill that illutrates the point is Cardizen R. I use it for example because it comes in the sizes 30mg, 60mg and 90mg.

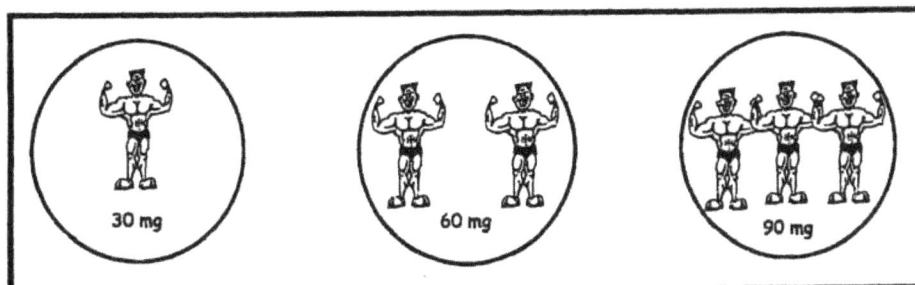

The 60mg pill is scored to easily split in two.

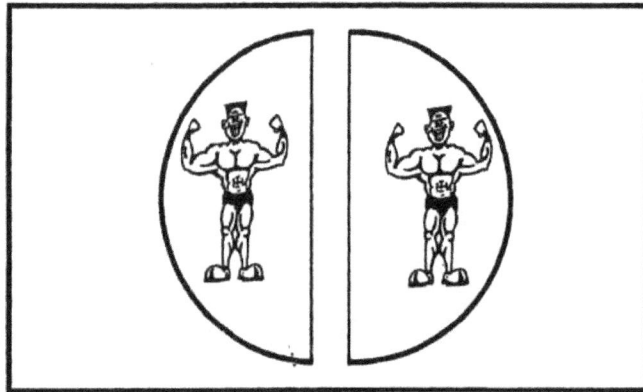

What if you needed 30mg and only had a 60mg pill?

The last pill that we'll talk about is scored so you can break it into thirds.  The anti depressant Desyrel 150mg is scored so it can be broken into thirds of 50mg each.

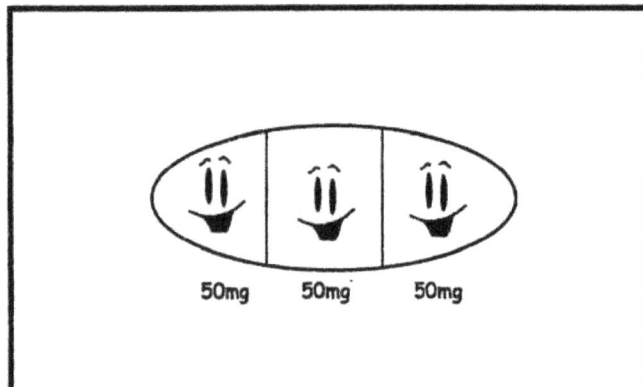

If the prescribed dose should be 100mg you would break off one part and give the other two.

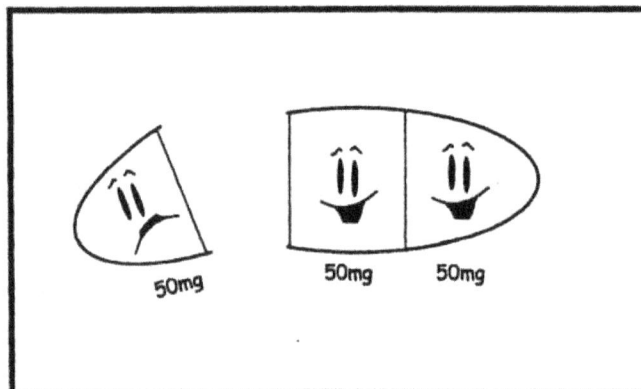

# CAPOTEN

Capoten is a blood pressure tablet that splits into four pieces. The whole tablet is 25mg.

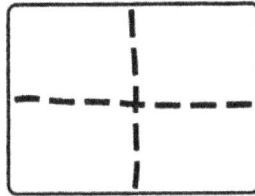

Until I wrote this book the square shape always seemed a little odd. But if you think about dividing anything into four equal parts I can see why. The whole tablet contains 25mg of active ingredients.

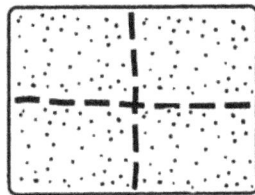

Suppose the order called for 12.5mg of Capoten, doesn't 1/2 of 25 equal 12.5?

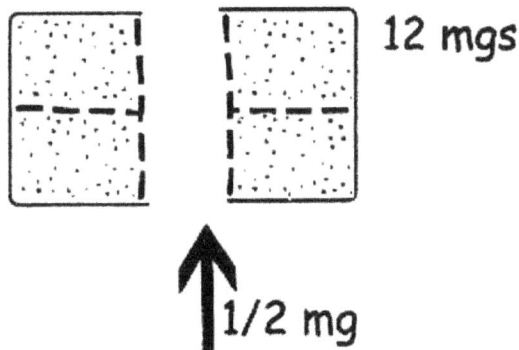

12 mgs

1/2 mg

Of course little milligrams are just shown for us to count as we split the pills. In reality the active ingredient is totally interspected throughout the pill.

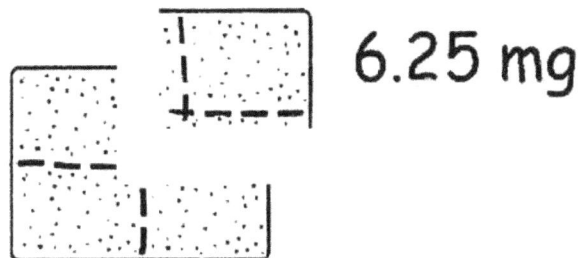

6.25 mg

Now suppose the doctor orders 6.25 mg of Capoten. Why would the doctor specify 6.25 mg? That's an odd number. Maybe that's because 6.25 is 1/4 of 25. Therefore 25 / 4 = 6.25

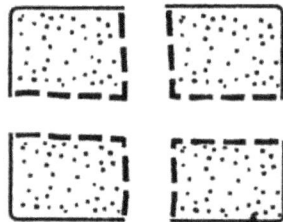

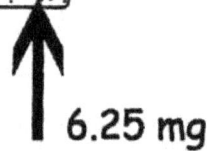

6.25 mg

INJECTABLE EXAMPLES

To begin injectable problems, the best example I can find is Ativan. It comes 2mg in a 2ml prefilled syringe.

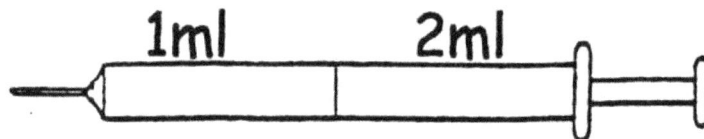

1ml          2ml

There is one mg of active ingredient in each ml.

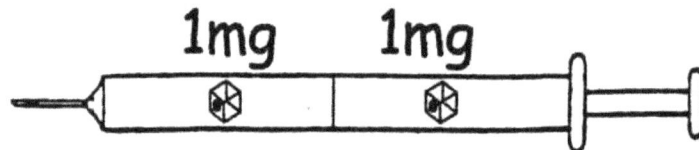

1mg          1mg

If you wanted (or rather the order called for) 1mg, you would inject 1ml.

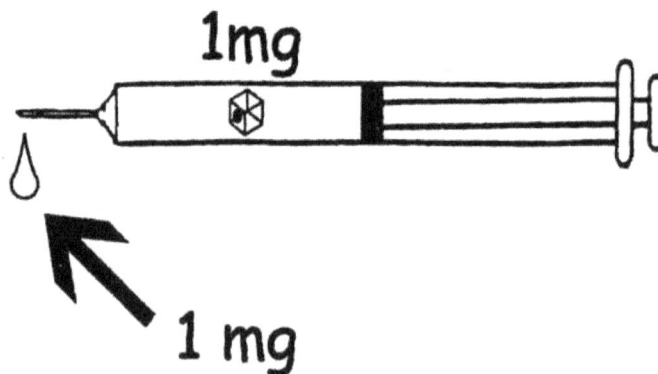

1mg

1 mg

Want to try more drugs? How about Tylenol Elixier liquid form. This is mostly for children who can't swallow pills. The mixture is 160mg of active ingredient in each 5cc. We'll be looking at how much Tylenol you'd give knowing how much Tylenol the patient needs.

First of all lets look at the quantities. 5ml is about one teaspoon.

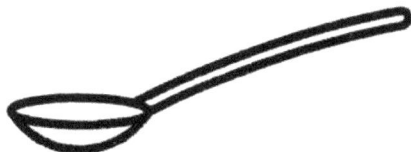

A typical child's dose would be given with a syringe. But for our purposes lets consider dosages from 160 to 1000mg, which are typical adult doses.

Let's start with 160mg. 160mg is a very small amount. You would need a magnifying glass and a tweezer to pick up this much of powder. But if we mix it up in a larger amount of liquid, we can measure and dispense it.

Probably you'd give an adult his Tylenol Elixir in a medicine cup and squirt it into an infant's mouth with a syringe. We'll use both methods in the next few examples.

O.K., 160mg in 5 ml that would be quick, either the 5ml mark on the medicine cup or the syringe. You might also notice that 5 ml is also marked one tsp on the syringe.

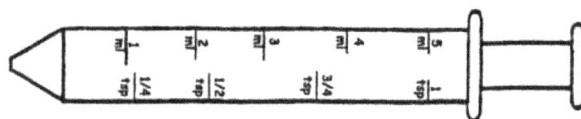

How about 80mg? How much Elixir would we pour or more likely for such a small amount squirt out of a syringe?

Half of the elixir (liquid) would give us half of the active ingredient.

1/2 of 5ml is 2 1/2ml

1/2 of 160ml is 80mg, which is what we want.

2.5ml
80 mg
Tylenol

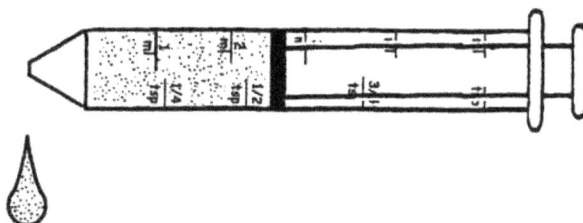

Lets take more of those situations of less than 5ml or 160mg.

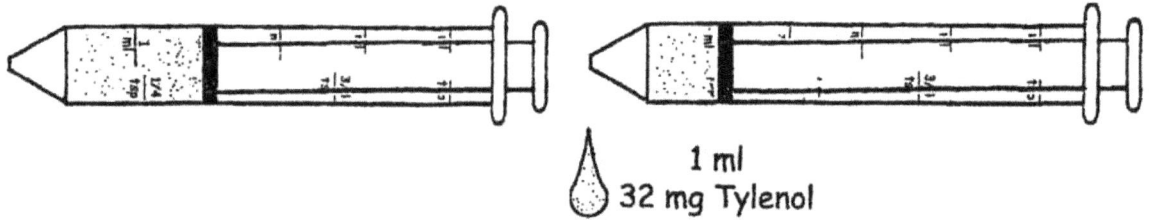

1 ml
32 mg Tylenol

Do you see the progression here. As we squirt out one milliliter we are also squirting out 32mg of active Tylenol. That's the whole point. That's always a good thoing to look for - how much active ingredient is in the smallest unit.

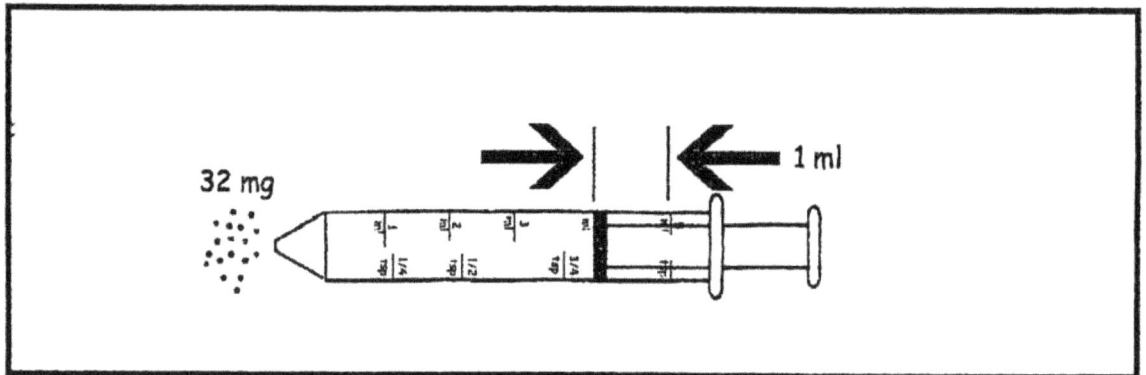

32 mg

1 ml

In this case we see that one ml contains 32mg and added together all 5ml coi tain 160mg. Which is what we were told originally.

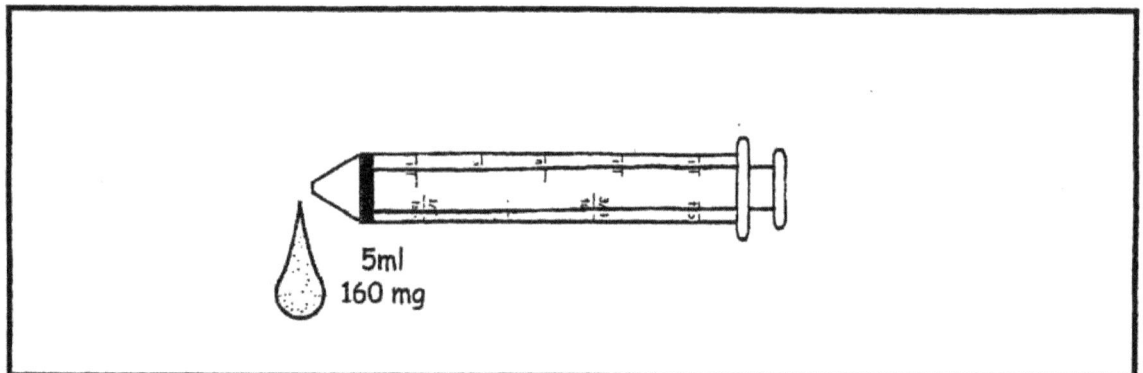

5ml
160 mg

Lets try another drug, injectable Demerol - the pain killer. Demerol is used for temporary moderate to severe pain, like fractures and surgical incisions. A typical adult gets 50 to 75mg. It comes in a prepacked syringe with 100mg in one ml.

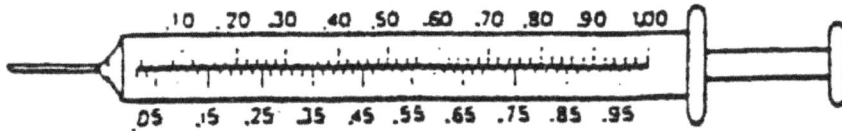

Lets work with this one for a while. We have gradually worked down the quantities from 5 gallons of Kool Aid to 2 tablespoons of coffee to 5ml of Tylenol Elixir to a 1ml injectable. Is that progress, or what??? You'll first notice how the syringe is marked.

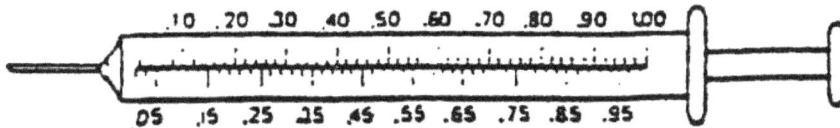

The unit we'll be dealing with to give the correct amount is 1/10 of a ml.

If we depressed the plunger to the first line we would squirt 1/10 of a milliliter. We would continue to squirt 1/10 ml each time we depressed the plunger past each line.

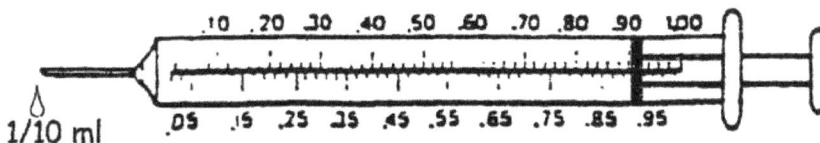

1/10 ml

Or we could squirt larger amounts by depressing the plunger a few 1/10ml lines at a time. Suppose we wanted to squirt five 1/10 or 5/10, which would give 50mg. We could depress the plunger past each 1/10 line 5 times.

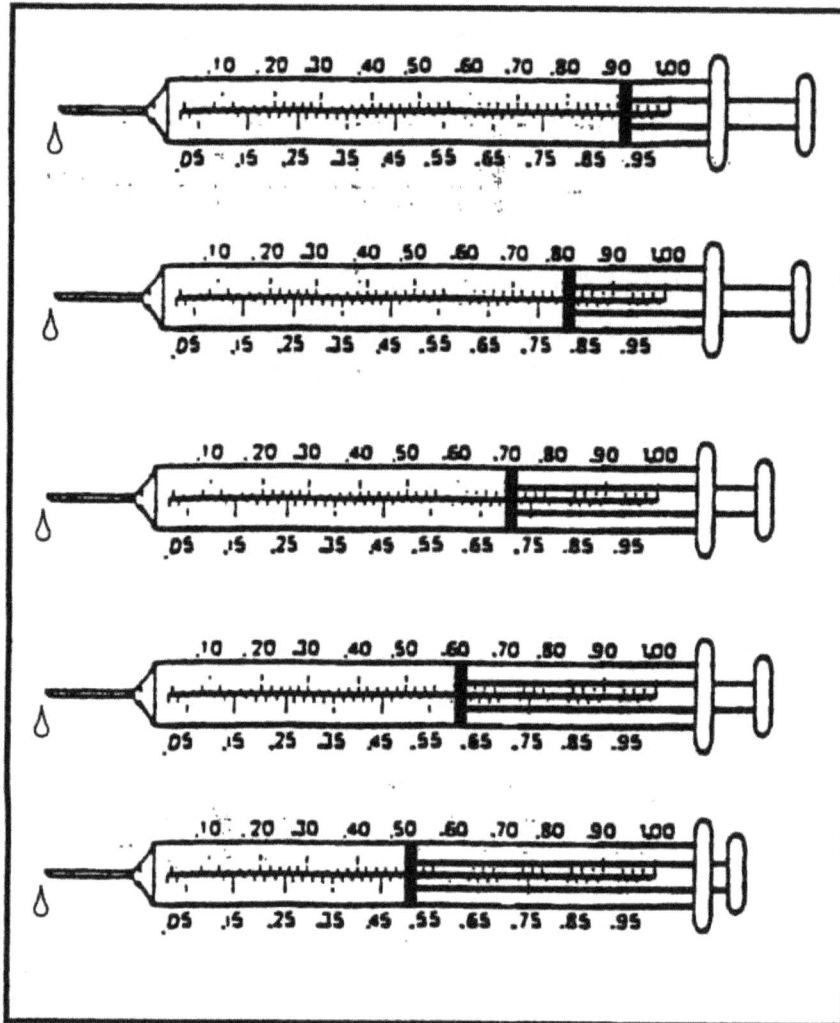

Or do it in one plunge.

Either way we would get 5/10 of a milliliter.

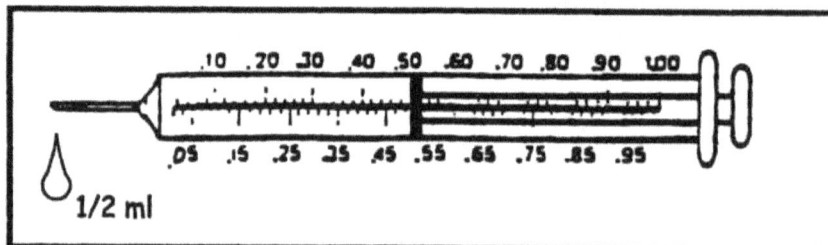

1/2 ml

Let's look at 1/4 of a milliliter. 1/4 in decimals is .25. What would .25 look like on our syringe? .25 is half way between .2 and .3.

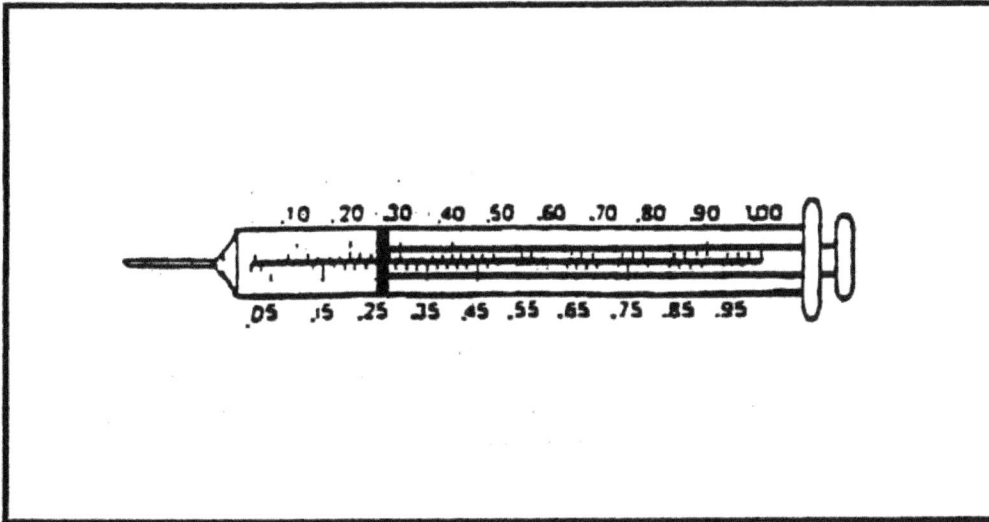

Lets look at .75. .75 is 3/4 on our syringe, .75 is half way between the .7 line and .8 line.

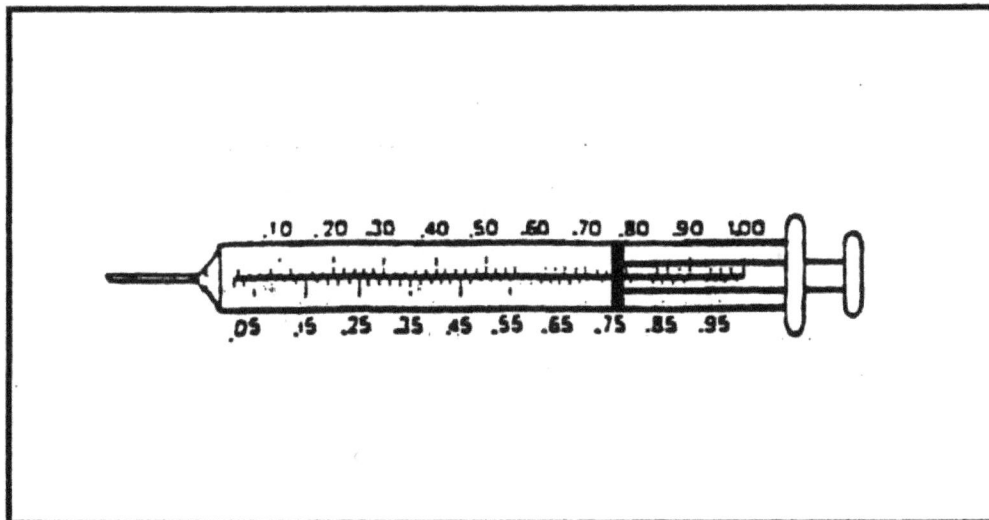

Are the fractions of a milliliter clear?

**Just say yes...**

Now lets look at how much active ingredient Demerol is in each of those tenths.

We said earlier that a paper clip weighs 500mg. That should give you an idea of how much the 100mg of true Demerol active ingredient weighs. Those 100mg are mixed evenly in the ml which is in our syringe.

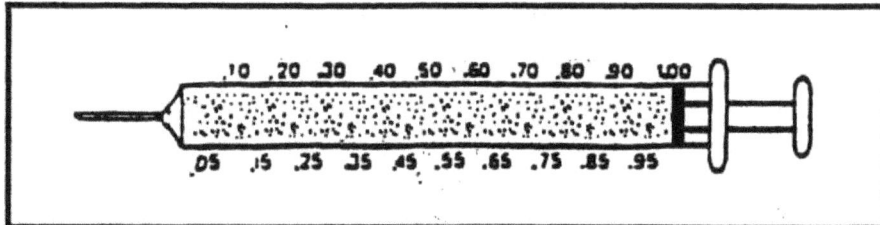

What we'll be doing next is very important. We will be figuring the injection quantity that complies with the doctor's order. There is one mg in each 1/100ml.

The doctor will prescribe a certain number of **milligrams**. Our job is to inject the correct number of **milliliters**.

Although the active ingredient is totally dissolved and invisible lets use this picture of 100mg of Demerol in a 1ml syringe.

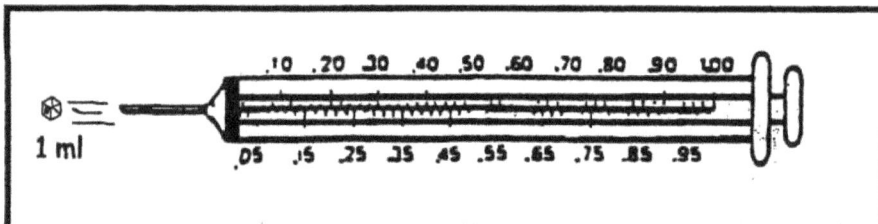

If the doctor orders 100mg we would depress the plunger enough to inject all 100mg or the whole ml. Ouch!!! Ahhh...

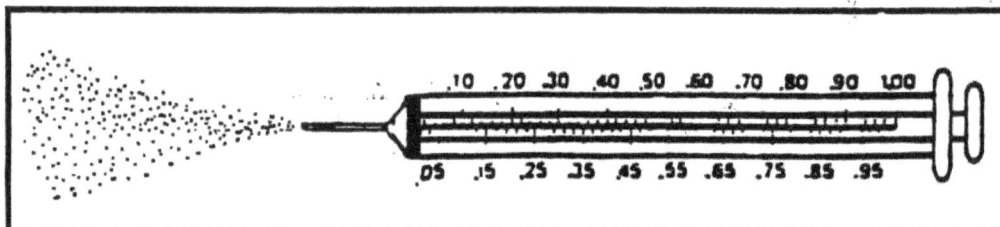

For the next few questions, just count the "visible" milligrams.
Soon you'll get the hang of it. Remember there is one mg in each 1/100ml, 10mg in each 1/10ml, 25mg in each 25/100 (or 1/4) ml.

Suppose the doctor ordered 50mg. We would first depress the plunger past each 1/10 line 5 times to eject 50mg, leaving 50mg to inject into the patient.

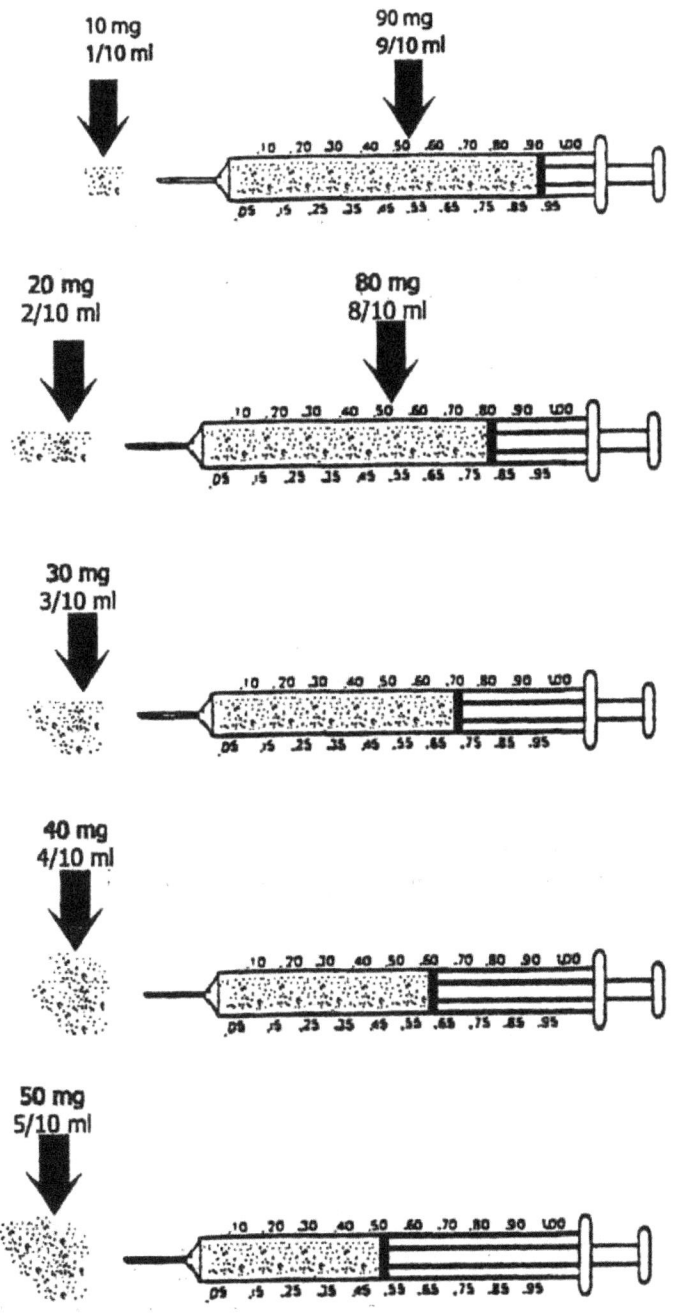

**10 mg**
**1/10 ml**

**90 mg**
**9/10 ml**

**20 mg**
**2/10 ml**

**80 mg**
**8/10 ml**

**30 mg**
**3/10 ml**

**40 mg**
**4/10 ml**

**50 mg**
**5/10 ml**

or do it in one plunge.

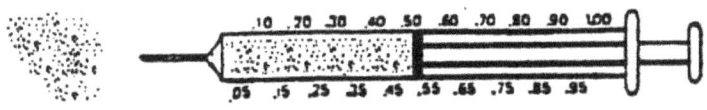

50mg left for injection.

Suppose the doctor ordered 80mg. We would discard 20mg by expelling 0.2ml. That would leave 0.8ml to inject.

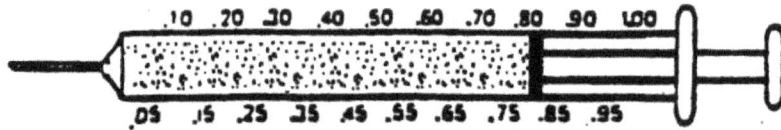

One more; suppose the doctor ordered 75mg. We would depress the plunger enough to expel 25mg which would leave 75mg. Lets look at the picture and count if we have to expelling 25mg would be little more than 2ml and a little less than 3ml. Even though 25ml is not clearly marked with a line, it can be easily estimated.

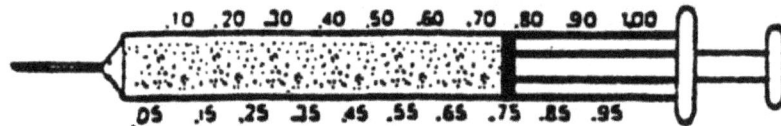

## Conclusion

Let's look at what we've been doing. We have been counting milligrams which are invisible by counting the milliliters which are clearly marked. We did this by knowing that there were 10mg in each 1/10ml. And from that we gave the right number of 1/10ml's.

# PRE-OP INJECTABLE EXAMPLE

I like these kind of examples because they are the most common "drug calcula-tions" that I see being done on a medical-surgical floor. They are especially important because three or four medications are calculated,"drawn up" and given under "pre op" conditions. In other words, when the O.R. is on the phone wanting to know "where is the patient?" The transporter is waiting outside the room with a stretcher. There are about six family members hanging over you. And you have to get and give the pre op medications and make sure the check list and the chart are complete. In other words, you'll be doing these calculations under less than ideal conditions.

Let's look at an order with three very frequently prescribed drugs-morphine, Versed and scopolamine. Morphine is a narcotic analgesic, a very strong pain reliever. Versed is a sedative. Scopolamine produces amnesia and decreases respiratory secre-tions. What we're going to do is individually squirt the three medications into one large syringe and put the needle on when we're done filling it. We'll chose from 3cc, 5cc and 10cc. Let's use a 5cc syringe.

The order calls for 0.4mg scopolamine, The scopolamine comes in a 1ml vial which contains 0.4mg of active ingredients. So we'll draw the whole ml and squirt it into the 5cc syringe.

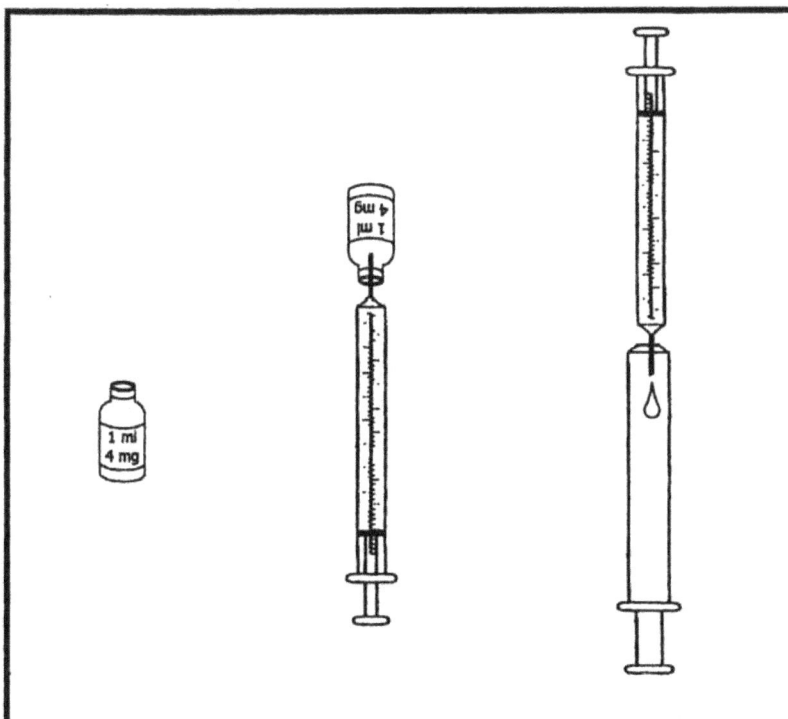

Versed comes 5mg in a 5ml vial. How many mg are in each ml?
There is one mg in each ml. So we will withdraw three ml and squirt them into the 5cc syringe

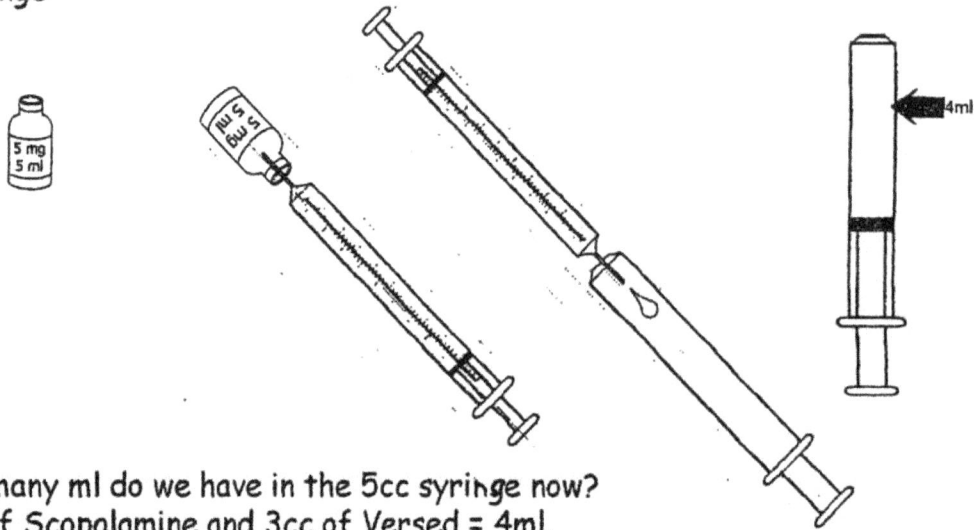

How many ml do we have in the 5cc syringe now?
1ml of Scopolamine and 3cc of Versed = 4ml.

Morphine comes in a prefilled 1ml syringe that contains 10mg of active ingredient Morphine Sulfate or MSO4. For ease of measuring the volume is marked in increments of 1/10ml. If there is one mg of
Morphine, how many 1/10s of a ml are there?

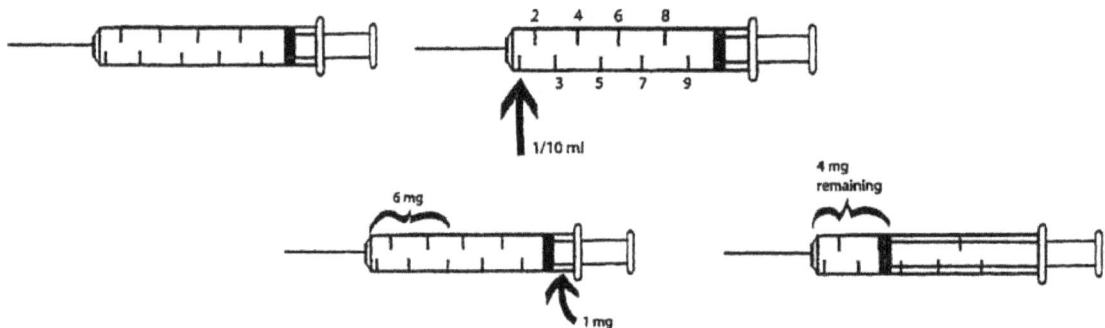

We want to add 6mg or 6 1/10s of a ml into our 5cc syringe.
That will leave .4ml ( 4 1/10s) in our Morphine syringe and
bring the volume to 4.6ml in our 5cc syringe. We would then
put a needle on and inject it into the patient.
1ml Scopolamine+3ml Versed+0.6 Morphine = 4.6 ml in our
5ml syringe. It's a good idea to check. Generally you
should limit an injection to 3ml. So in this case you
would divide the injection into two syringes. One
with 3ml and one with 1.6ml or more evenly
2.3ml in each syringe.

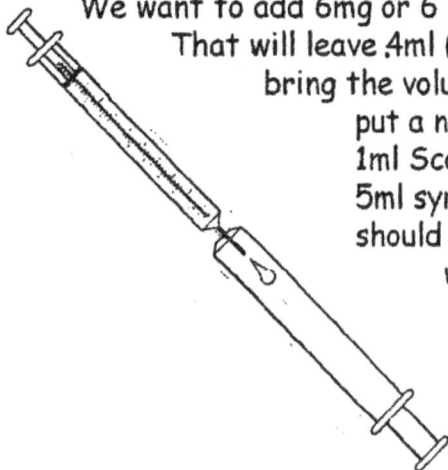

Lets look at a real life situation. A very typical order before surgery might read:

1 gm Ancef
6 mg MS
3mg versed
0.3 mg Scopolamine
10 mg Reglan

I.M.

I.M. of course means intra muscular, an injection.

Ancef    (cefazolin) is a broad spectrum antibiotic. A good lesson that you'll need to remember as long as you're a nurse is **Never Mix** an antibiotic with any other medication. So you would not mix anything with the Ancef.

Ancef comes as a powder in a vial. The directions say add 2.5ml of sterile water. Sterile water is just what it claims to be sterile water. It is used for reconstituting powders.

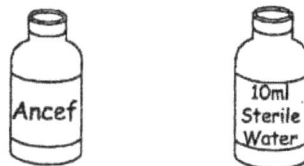

Then inject the water into the vial and make sure the liquid is clear. Withdraw the reconstituted Ancef in the same syringe and label it with tape "Ancef 1 gram."

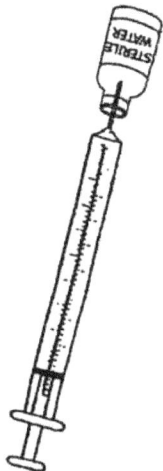

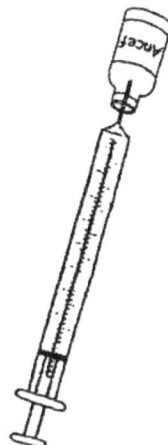

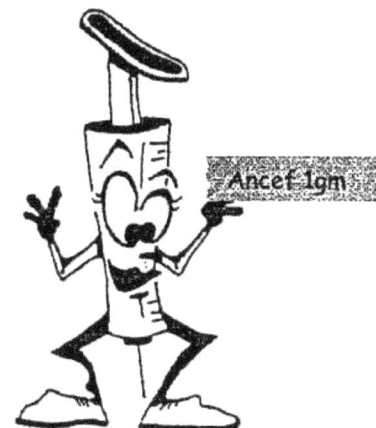

Before you start to draw up the other medications write the label for the next syringe. It will read:

M.S.  6mg
Versed 3mg
Scopolamine 0.3mg
Reglan 10mg

That's a lot to write on one tape. But it will avoid a mistake. I would write it on a piece of 3" tape.

Ms  6mg
Versed  3mg
Scopolamine  0.3mg
Reglan  10mg

The next step is to get the morphine sulfate (M.S.) and versed. They are narcotics and would certainly be locked and require a count and signature to remove. The Scopolamine and Reglan would probably be in the patient's medication drawer or the general stock in the medication room.

What we are going to do is draw up the correct amount from each vial and squirt them into one syringe (one injection with four medications).

Lets look at the size of the syringe we'll need. We have 3cc, 5cc and 10cc syringes. Which ever one we use, we'll squirt the medications into it and put a needle on.

Lets estimate the volume we need.

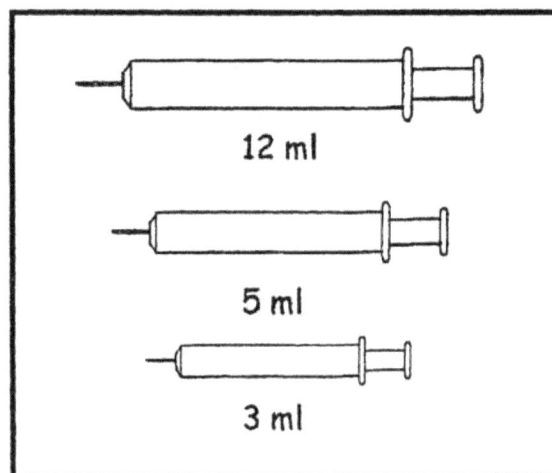

12 ml

5 ml

3 ml

The whole morphine vial is 1ml. We need less than the whole vial or less than one ml.

From the bottle of Scopolamine .4mg is 1ml. Once again we need less than the whole vial or less than one ml.

10mg of Reglan is 1ml. We need the whole vial or one ml.

Versed is 5mg in 5ml and we need 3mg Which is 3ml

By quickly estamating the volume we need about 5ml. So it wouldn't hurt to use a larger 10cc syringe.

Let's start with the Versed. The vial reads 5mg for 5ml. How many ml would we need to draw? We'll draw 3cc and squirt them into the 10cc syringe.

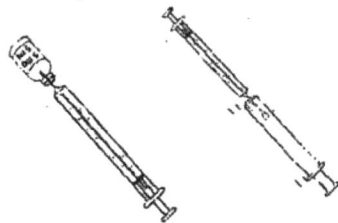

Next is Scopolamine which comes in a 1ml vial containing 0.4mg.
The vial says 0.4mg per ml and we need 0.3mg. For less than 1cc I would use a 1cc tuberculin syringe. Then as before squirt it into the 10cc syringe. Now the 10cc syringe we've been filling contains _____cc?

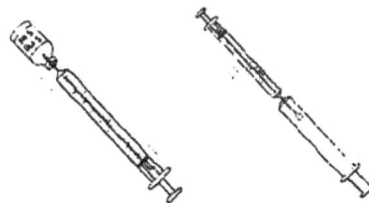

Moving right along. The Reglan vial says 10mg per ml and we need 10mg. So we need 1ml or the whole contents of the vial.

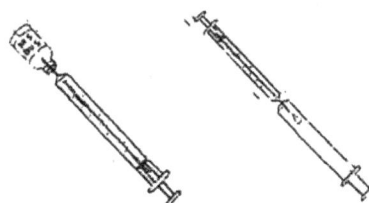

Last the Morphine.

Morphine comes in a prefilled syringe with 10mg in 1ml.

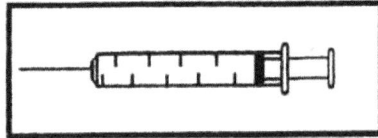

The order calls for 6mg. The syringe will always be clearly marked in 1/10 increments.

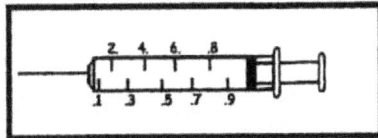

How much should we squirt into the syringe we're filling. One milliliter has 10 tenths of a milliliter. Each line is a tenth of a milliliter.

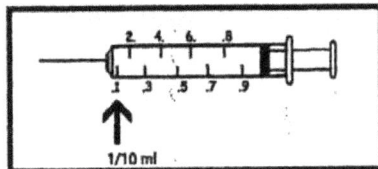

Each whole ml has 10mg. Each tenth ml has 1 mg.

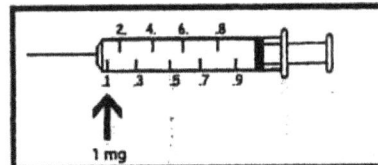

Since the 10mg of Morphine is completly dissolved in the milliliter of solution, we know that each tenth of the total volume contains 1mg of the Morphine. So to get 6mg we would squirt 6/10ml into our syringe.

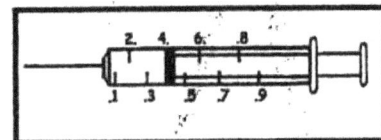

How much have we squirted in so far?
   1ml Reglan
   0.75ml Scopolamine
   3ml Versed
   0.6ml Morphine

You should verify a volume of 5.35ml in our 10cc syringe.Generally you would limit an injection to 3ml. So you would divide this into 3ml and 2.35ml.

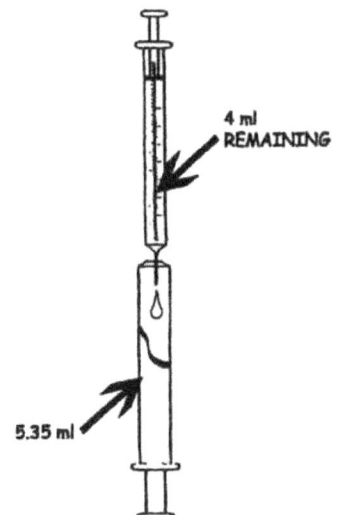

# I.V. DRIP RATE CALCULATIONS

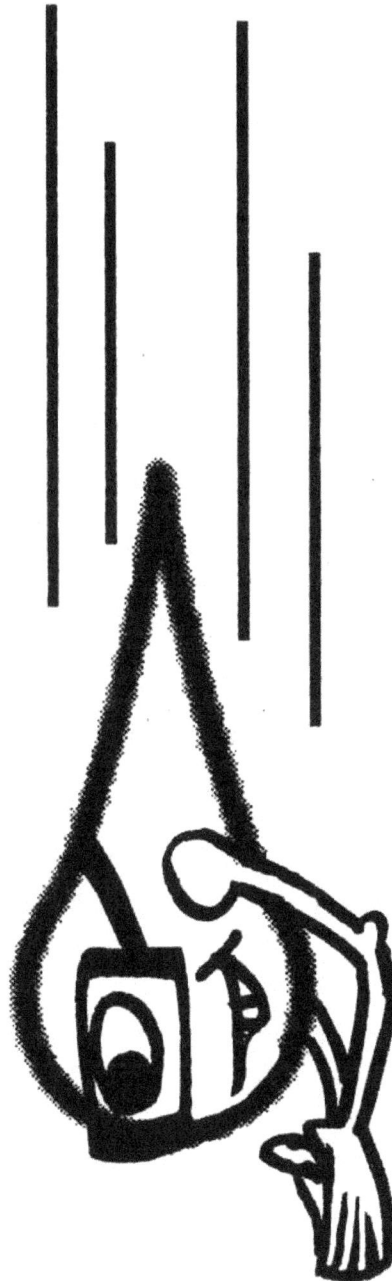

# Memorization

You may not belive this, but, **Memorizing** these four definitions will enable you to do IV calculations while you are **learning them**.

1.)"Flow Rate is the amount of fluid that flows per unit of time (cc per minute)"

2.)"Drip Rate is the number of drops per minute (gtt/min)"

3.)"Drop Factor is the number of drops per cubic centimeter (gtt/cc)"

4.)"Flow Rate = Drip Rate divided by Drop Factor and I want the Drip Rate"

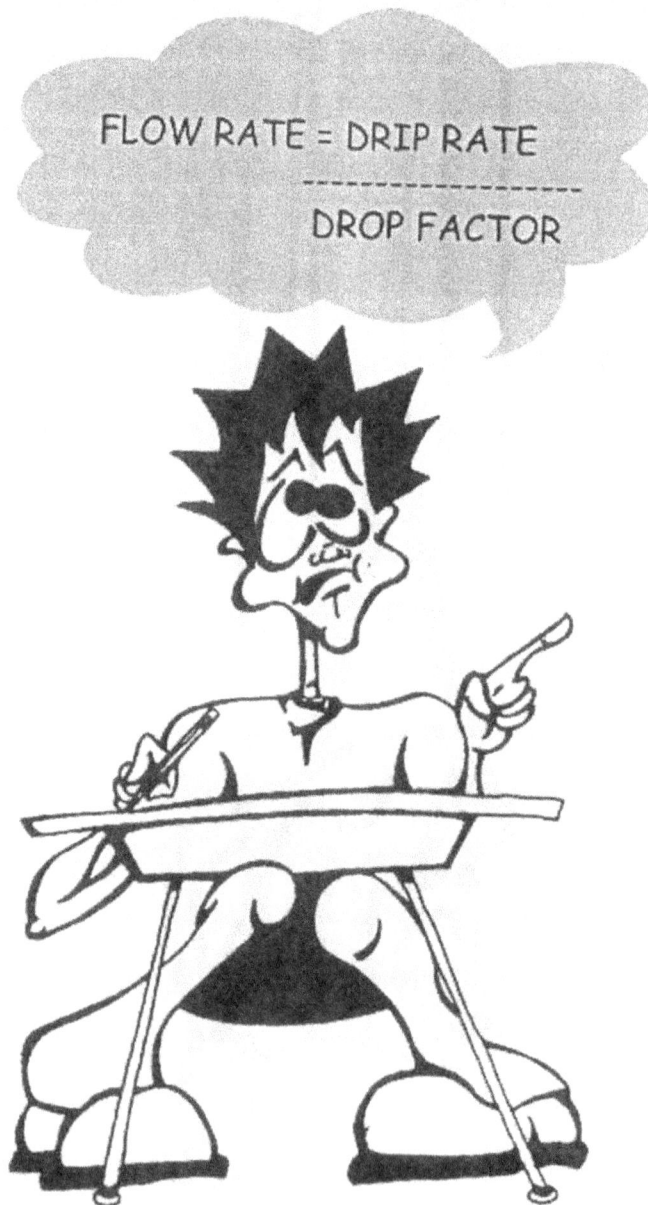

$$\text{FLOW RATE} = \frac{\text{DRIP RATE}}{\text{DROP FACTOR}}$$

## Flow Rate

There are a few simple terms that we will learn about.  The first is "Flow Rate."

You could say Flow Rate is how fast the fluid is flowing.  For example, on a larger scale, lets look at the faucet on your sink.  Turn the water on normally and it might take 15 seconds to fill a glass.  A typical drinking glass is a little more than 10 oz. or 320ml.  So the Flow Rate of your faucet is 320ml in 15 seconds, or 22ml/sec.  Now turn the water on full blast and it takes maybe 5 seconds and the Flow Rate is 64ml/sec.  Last, turn it all the way down to just the smallest trickle.  In my sink it took 5 1/2 minutes and the Flow Rate is 76ml/min. - as always the quantity divided by the time it took.

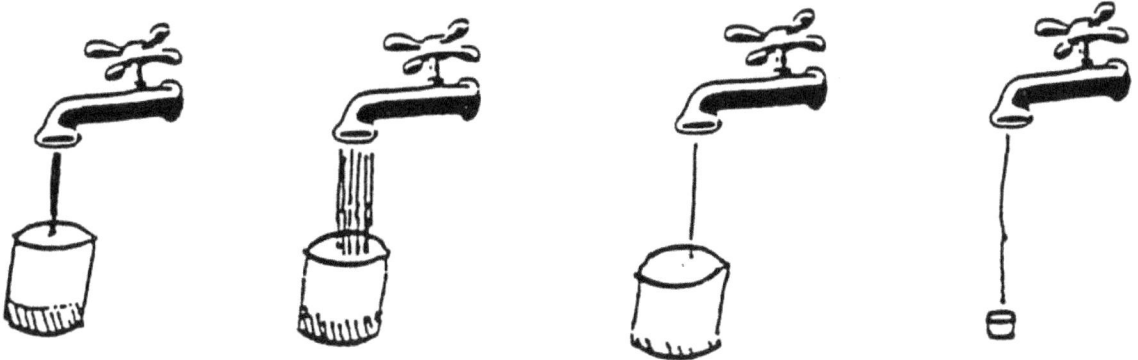

$$\frac{320ml}{15sec} = \frac{22ml}{sec}$$

$$\frac{320ml}{5sec} = \frac{64ml}{sec}$$

$$\frac{320ml}{330sec} = \frac{1ml}{sec}$$
(not quite,
but almost
1ml/sec)

$$\frac{30ml}{30sec} = \frac{1ml}{sec}$$

Lets turn the faucet to its smallest stream and see how long it takes to fill the 30cc container.  My sink took 30 seconds.  The smallest Flow Rate of my faucet is 30cc in 30 seconds or 1cc/sec.

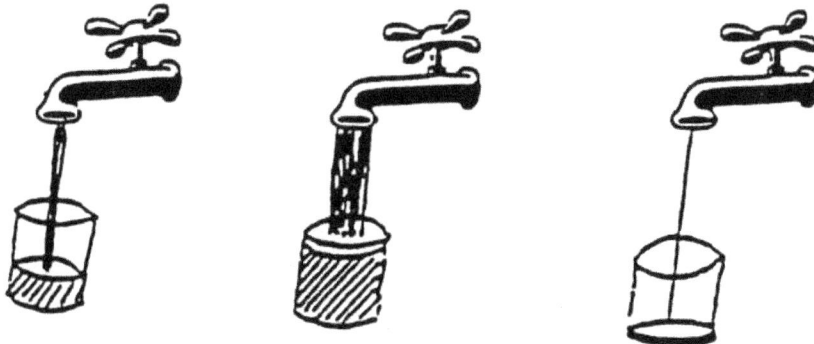

If we were to run the faucet for 5 seconds the first glass would be about 1/3 full, the second, with the faucet wide open would fill up, and the smallest stream would barely cover the bottom of the glass.

normal flow   $\dfrac{22ml}{sec} = \dfrac{1320ml}{min} = \dfrac{79,200ml}{hour}$   1½ 55gal drum

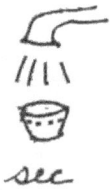

sec

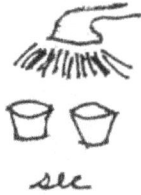

min

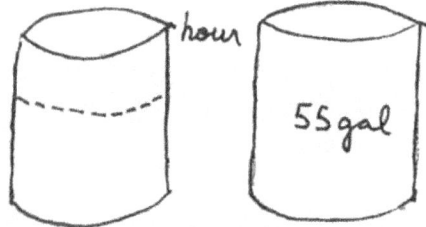

wide open   $\dfrac{64ml}{sec} = \dfrac{3840ml}{min} = \dfrac{230,400ml}{hour}$   about 4 55gal drum

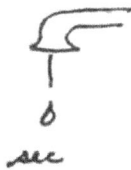

sec

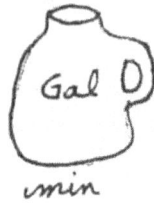

min

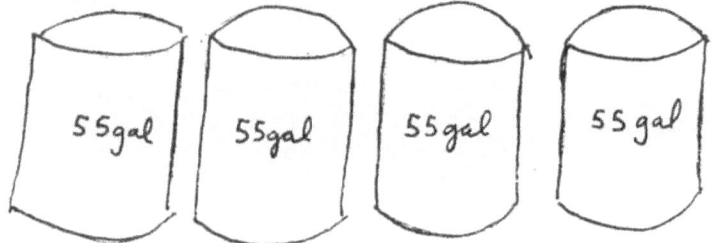

a trickle   $\dfrac{1ml}{sec} = \dfrac{60ml}{min} = \dfrac{3600ml}{hour}$

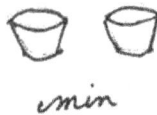

min

sec

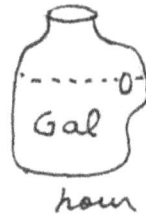

Gal

hour

normal IV flowrate   $83\dfrac{ml}{hour}$

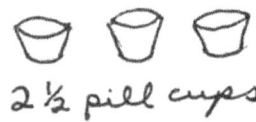

2½ pill cups - abou

$150\dfrac{ml}{hour}$

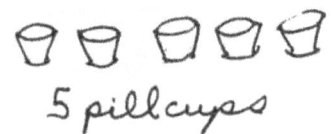

5 pill cups

Another concept in Flow Rate is converting units from seconds to minutes to hours. You can also try this in your faucet, although it would waste a little water, (that's O.K., just add 30ml Scotch and drink it when you are done.)

The "Normal Flow," 22ml/sec, is 1320ml/min or a little more than a quart a minute. Full blast, wide open 3840ml/min would fill almost 4 quarts in a minute. The smallest flow 1ml/sec would fill two pill cups, 60cc, in a minute.

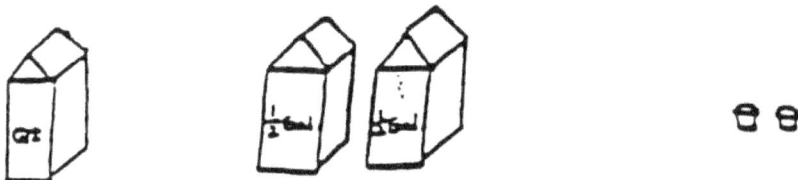

Going to those Flow Rates expressed in hours, your kitchen faucet would fill a 55 gallon drum in an hour and the slowest Flow Rate, 3600cc about 1 gallon.

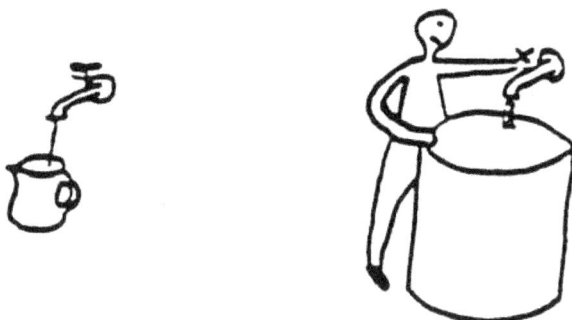

30cc in 30 seconds is 1cc per second. In one minute or 60 seconds we would have 60cc. The rate is 60cc per minute. How about the same Flow rate per hour, if 60cc flow in one minute and there are 60 minutes in an hour, then the same Flow Rate is 3600cc per hour. That's 3.6 liters or about 3 1/2 quarts. (On second thought if you do try this in your sink, don't add Scotch and drink it - not the hourly one anyway.)

Do you see the concept here:

$$\frac{30cc}{30 \text{ sec}} = \frac{1cc}{sec} = \frac{60cc}{min} = \frac{3600cc}{hr}$$

We have shown the same Flow Rate in terms of seconds, minutes and hours. That's because the doctor's orders may call for IV Flow Rate in hours and you have to convert that into something you can work with, like minutes.

## Flow Rate Example

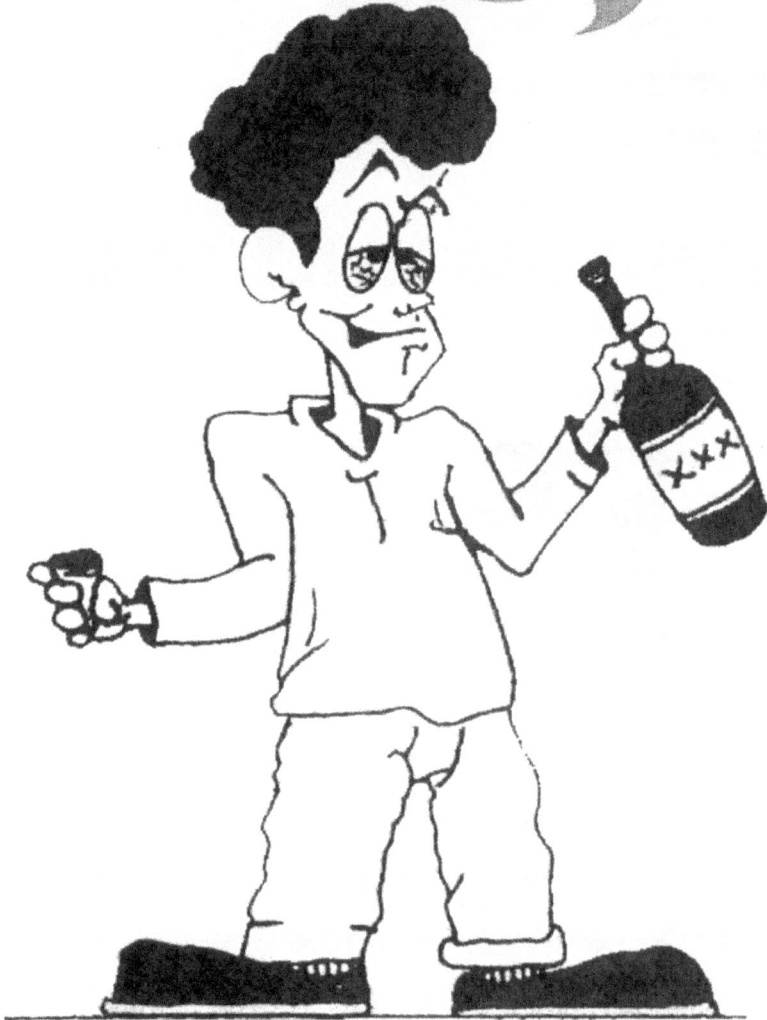

Lets try another Flow Rate conversion example. Suppose your sink faucet filled up a 30cc container in 45 seconds. What would the Flow Rate be in seconds, minutes and hours? For seconds the Flow Rate is 30cc per 45 seconds or 30cc/45 sec=.67cc/sec.

Because there are 60 seconds in a minute if we waited one minute there would be 60x.67cc flowing in a minute or 40cc/minute.

If we let the sink run for an hour we would get 60 times the amount in a minute or 2400cc/hour.

How about working the other way, since doctor's often give orders in liters and hours. 3000cc/hour, How much per minute?

There are 60 minutes in an hour. So the same Flow Rate would be 3000/60 or 50cc/minute

## Another Flow Rate Example

Determine the Flow Rate of an IV infusion if the doctor ordered "1000ml to be given in 12 hours." First of all notice the phrase "Flow Rate." Remember the defintion. We haven't gotten to drops yet so don't freak out.

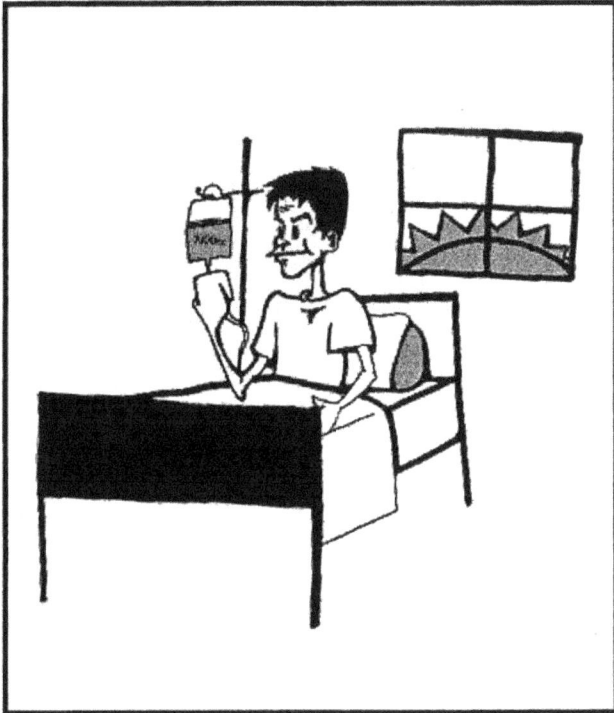

After one hour has passed, it is 10:00. How many cc's have flowed?

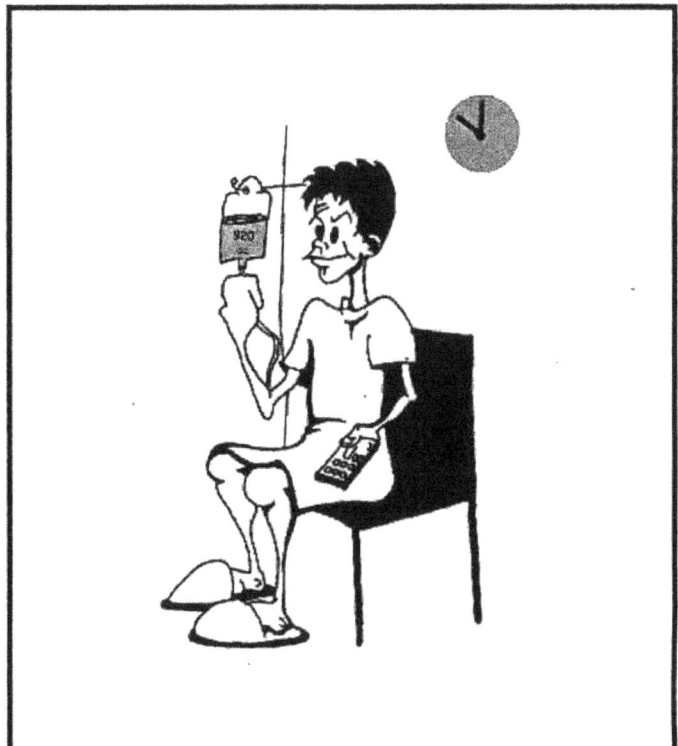

After two hours have passed,
how many cc's have flowed?

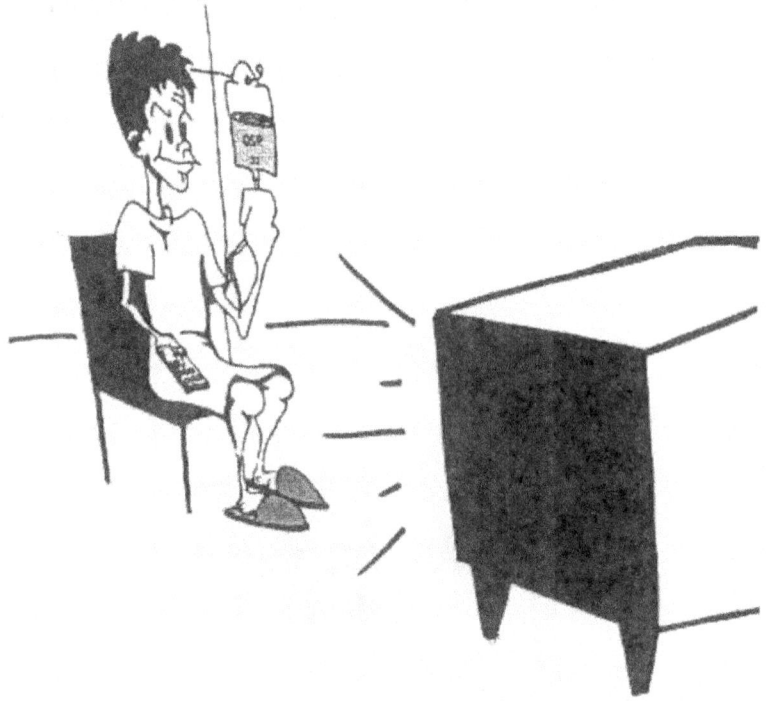

At lunch time (a little late) 1:00pm 332cc
have flowed. To keep this from being X-rated, I
didn't draw in the foley but about how full do you
think it would be?
(Hint: trick question, notice the **cup** on his tray).

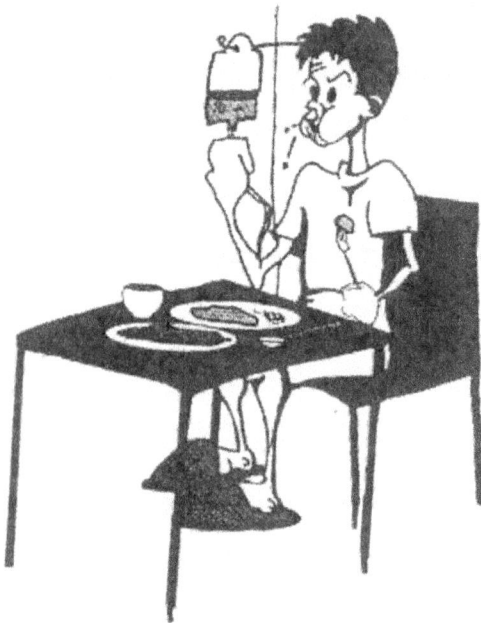

At 8:59 or 20:59 the whole liter has
just about finished and his nurse will
discontine the IV.

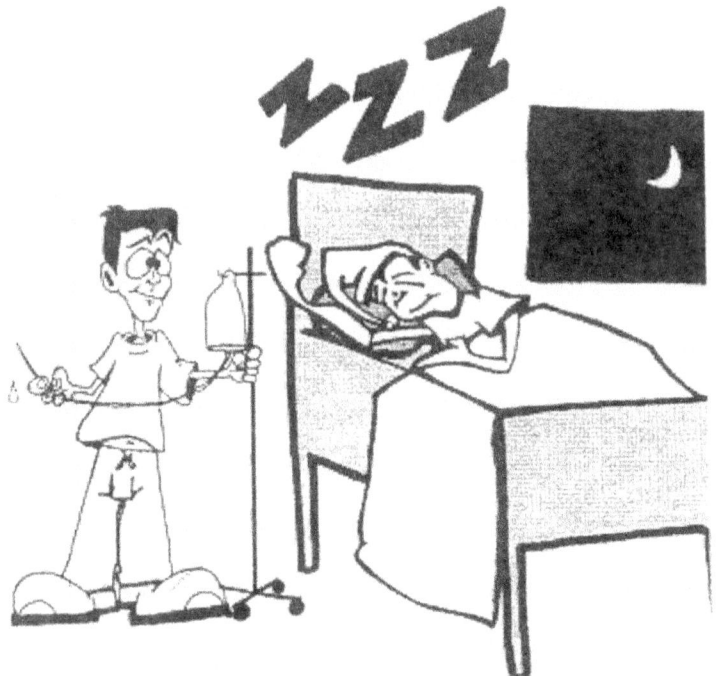

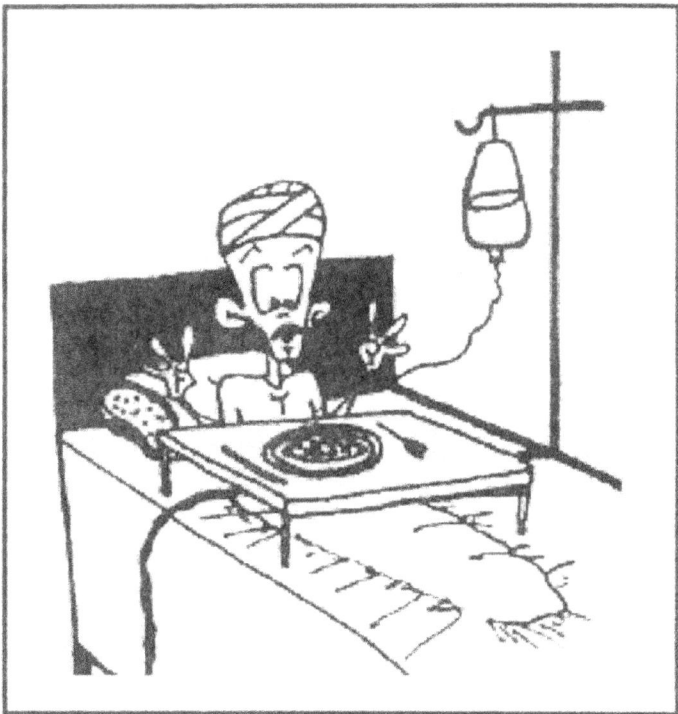

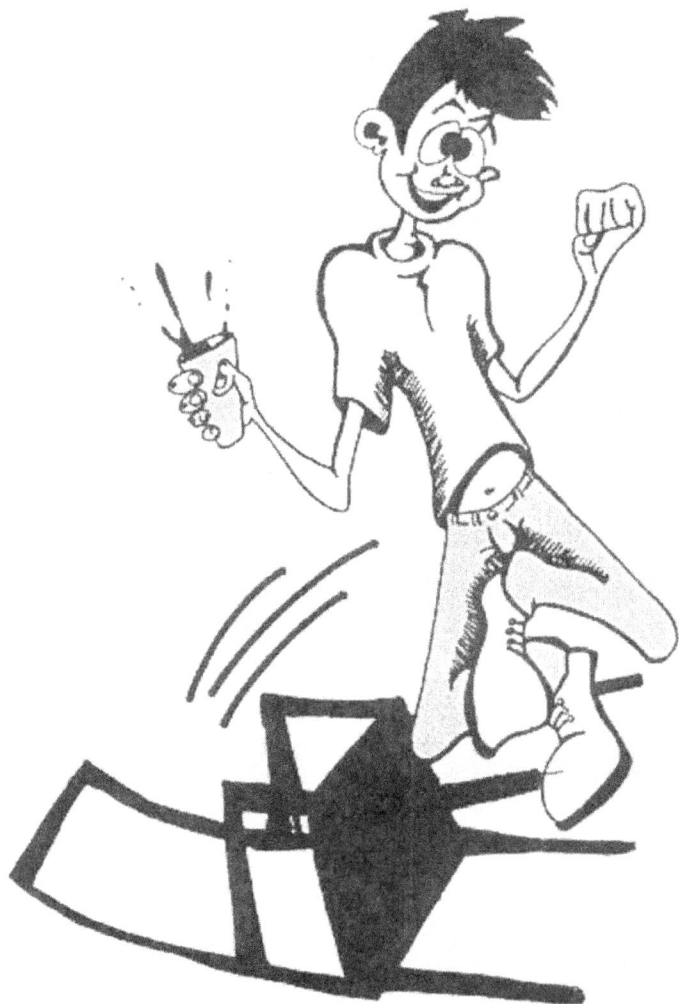

ALRIGHT!

# I.V. Technique

I'm jumping ahead slightly here. We're going to learn a technique that you will definitely use in any hospital setting.

If our patient in the last problem was on an IV drip a problem could have occurred - the Drip Rate might change. If you remember the anatomy of an IV you'll understand.

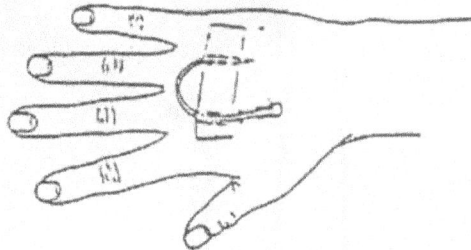

A very thin, very flexible tube is "threaded" into a vein, The "invasion" of the vein is only possible because the tube is so very thin and flexible. But a look at its size shows how any motion of a relatively huge arm could bend or compress and occlude the tube. This is called "positional" - meaning very sensitive to position.

You can imagine that the patient would have moved his arm in the twelve hour running time. And any change in position would affect the Flow Rate. To make sure the flow doesn't deviate too much from our plan we will label the bag with hours next to the volume we'd expect at that time. We do this by putting a piece of tape along the length of the bag and marking the expected time next to the volume.

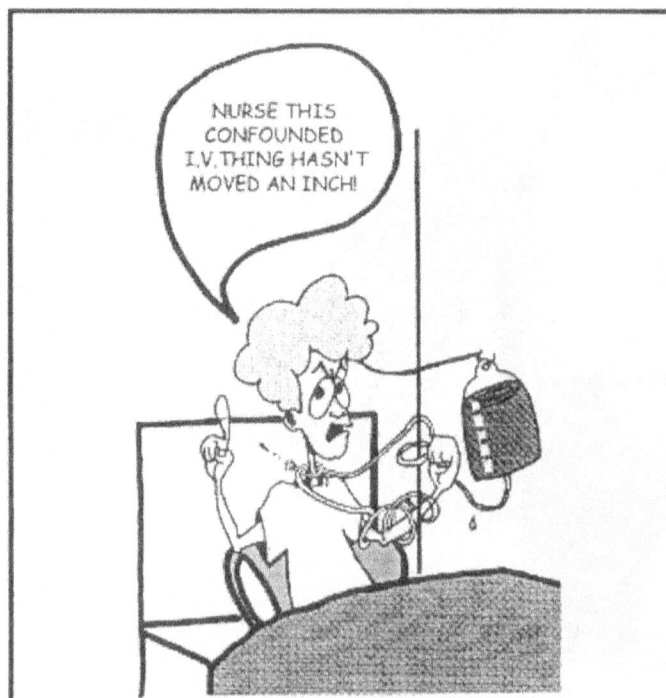

If the order was 1000cc in 12 hours we determined that in the first hour 83cc should have flowed. That would leave 917cc in the bag. 10:00 just a little above the 900cc line. At 11:00 166cc are supposed to have dripped leaving 834. We would mark 11:00 as nearly as possible to that volume on the bag. We would mark the bag incrementally for the next 12 hours. We do this by subtracting 83cc from the volume at the last hour. This way you could pop in the room, look at your watch, look at the bag and know right away if its flowing correctly.

There are many ways he could have occluded the flow temporarily or permanently. He could have rolled over on the tube, or more likely by just moving his arm, tightened the muscles and slowed down the flow. You will be able to see this if the volume is lagging the time next to it.

To get around this problem Pumps have come into common usage. They "Pump" the fluid at whatever rate you set. Whenever the pump senses a decrease in flow (for any of the numerous reasons mentioned) they will alarm. For this reason you don't have to mark the bag - the pump tells you exactly how much has flowed. And if it hasn't beeped too often the rate should be close to what you'd expect.

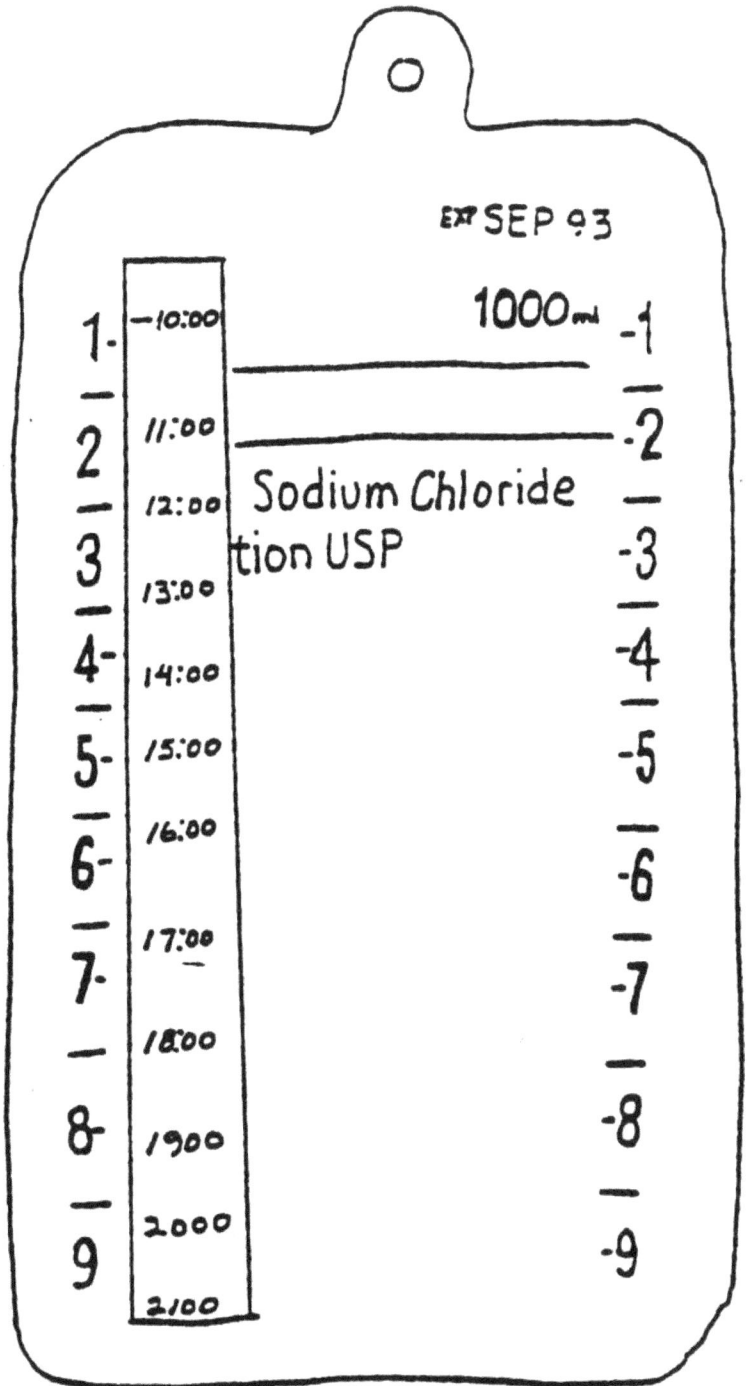

EXP SEP 93

1000 ml

1-
2-
3-
4-
5-
6-
7-
8-
9-

10:00
11:00
12:00
13:00
14:00
15:00
16:00
17:00
18:00
1900
2000
2100

Sodium Chloride
tion USP

-1
-2
-3
-4
-5
-6
-7
-8
-9

# DROP FACTOR

Drop Factor is quite simple (yeah..right). There are only two things to know:

1.) When fluid slowly flows out of small holes it comes out in drops - not a stream.

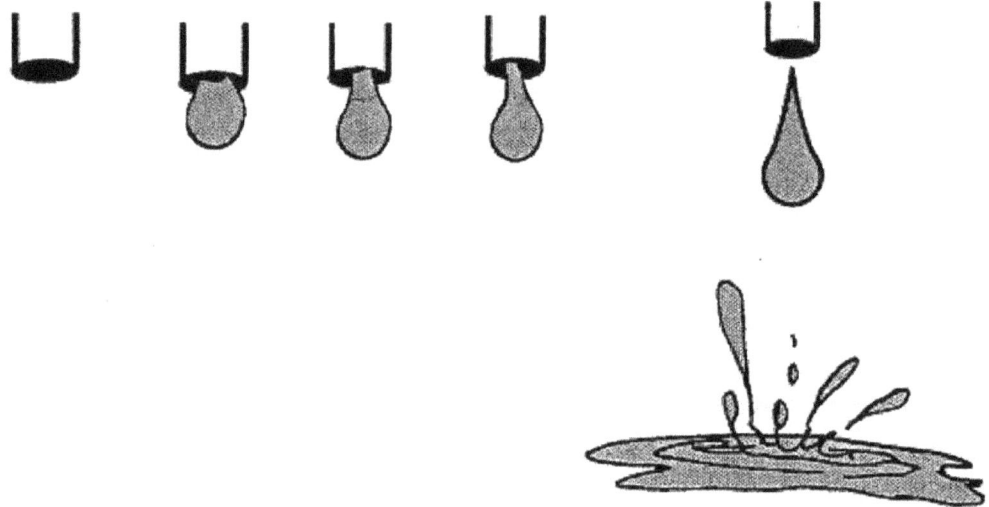

2.) For each hole size those drops are always the same. Small drops come out of small holes and big drops come out of big holes.

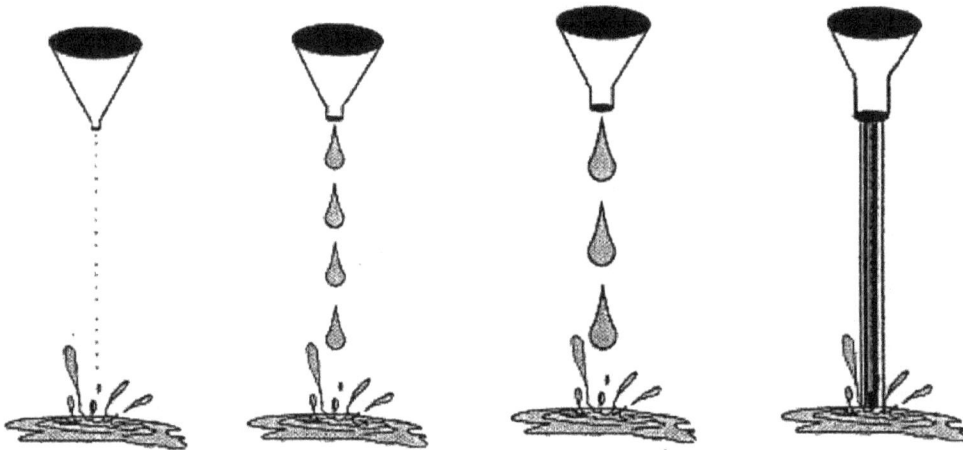

If the hole gets too big a stream comes out. You can visualize this by turning down your faucet till the small stream becomes an annoying drip. Since the size of each drop is the same we express this size as its volume, drops per ml (gtt/ml), or Drop Factor.

If you cognitive mind rejected everything I just said, this example has got to stick. In fact it's so good you could skip the rest of the book - which is why I didn't mention it earlier.

Step #1. Take a small syringe 3 to 5cc.

Step #2. Take a few different needles from 18 gage to 25 gage.

Step #3 .With the largest needle in place draw up exactly 1cc of water.

Step #4. Gently & Slowly tap down the plunger while you count the number of drops it takes to deplete exactly 1cc.

Step #5,6. Take diffrent needles and repeat. Is that the Drop Factor?
      (Hint: yes, it is.)

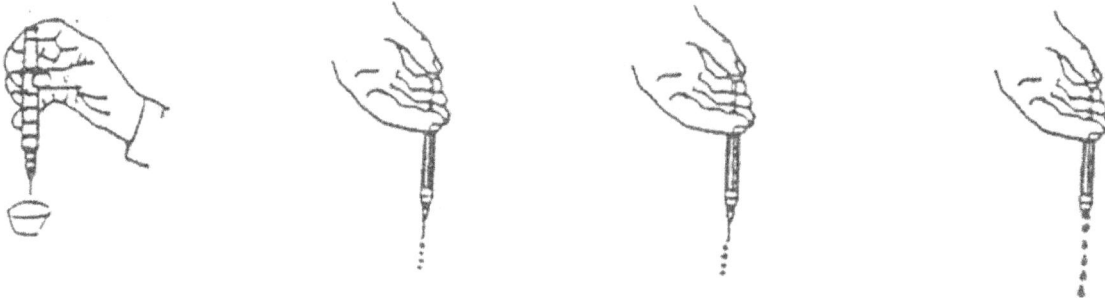

     I got 145 gtt/cc for the 25 gage needle & 60 gtt/cc for the 18 gage. Then I took the needle off, filled the syringe, let the water drop out and found that it took 18 drops to deplete 1cc.

Do you see how counting drops can be the same as counting cc's. And setting the Drip Rate in drops per minute (gtt/min) is the same as setting the Flow Rate in cc's per minute (cc/min)

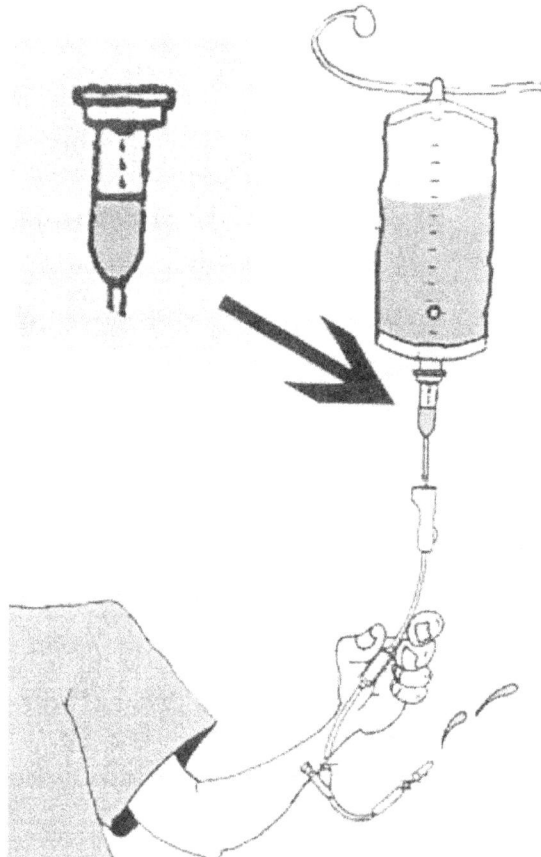

In practical situations all IV tubing looks like this:

The sharp end of the tubing punctures the bag. Just below the bag is the drip chamber.

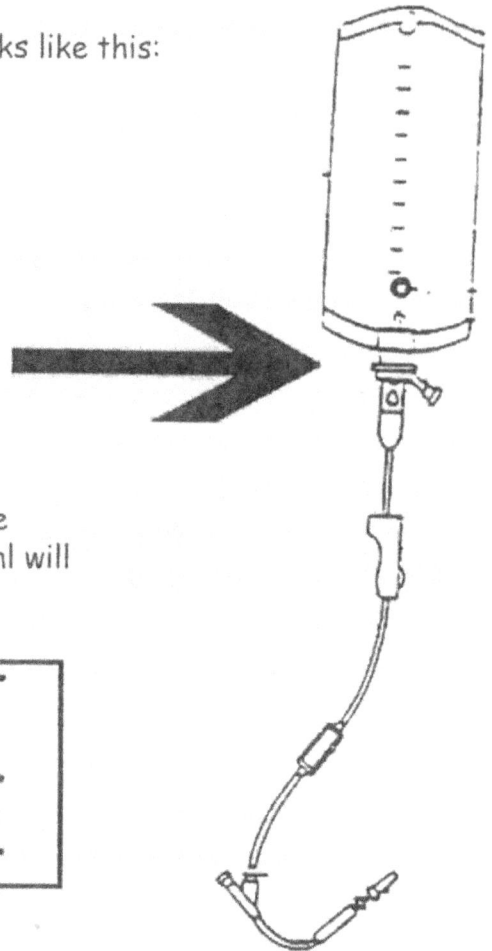

In the drip chamber the fluid drips out a needle where you can watch it. The number of drops/ml will always be marked clearly on the box.

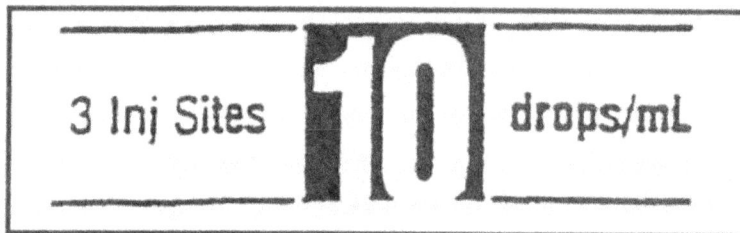

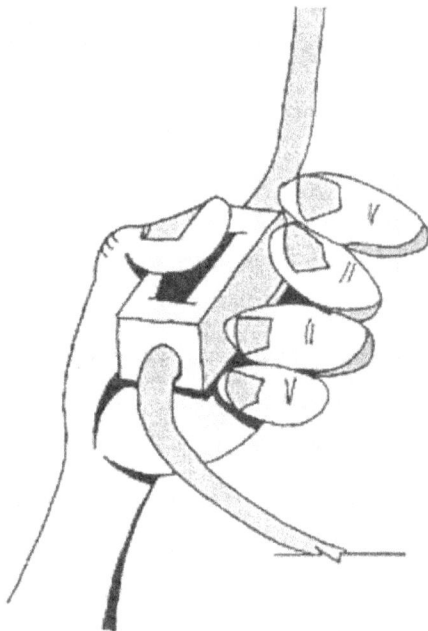

3 Inj Sites **10** drops/mL

Knowing the Drop Factor enables you to set the IV to the ordered Flow Rate. You do this by pinching the tubing with a roller clamp.

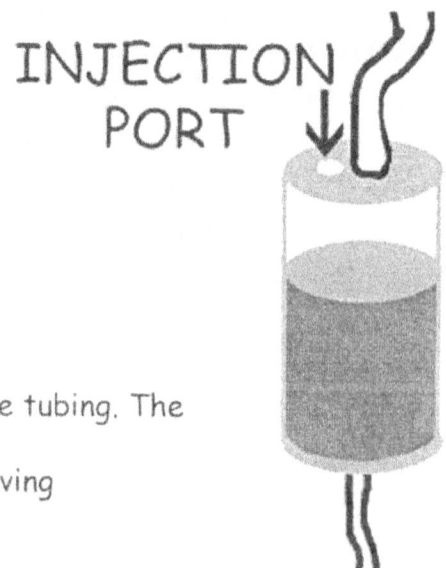

INJECTION PORT

A Buritrol is a container that can be connected to the tubing. The ports allow medications to be added to the IV infusion at specific times. This is much easier than giving the patient a "shot".

CONVERSION

At this point we understand Flow Rate and Drop Factor. Those are always given in the doctor's orders and whatever IV tubing you use. What we want is the Drip Rate.

I think the best way to solve for the Drip Rate is to use the equation:

**Flow Rate = Drip Rate/DropFactor**

I know that is algebra and most of you hate algebra. However, this books simplifies it to the level of multiplication. The only thing you must do is:

1.) change the units into ml and minutes.
2.) mulitiply

Lets first try to grasp this physically. To say the equation is a picture:

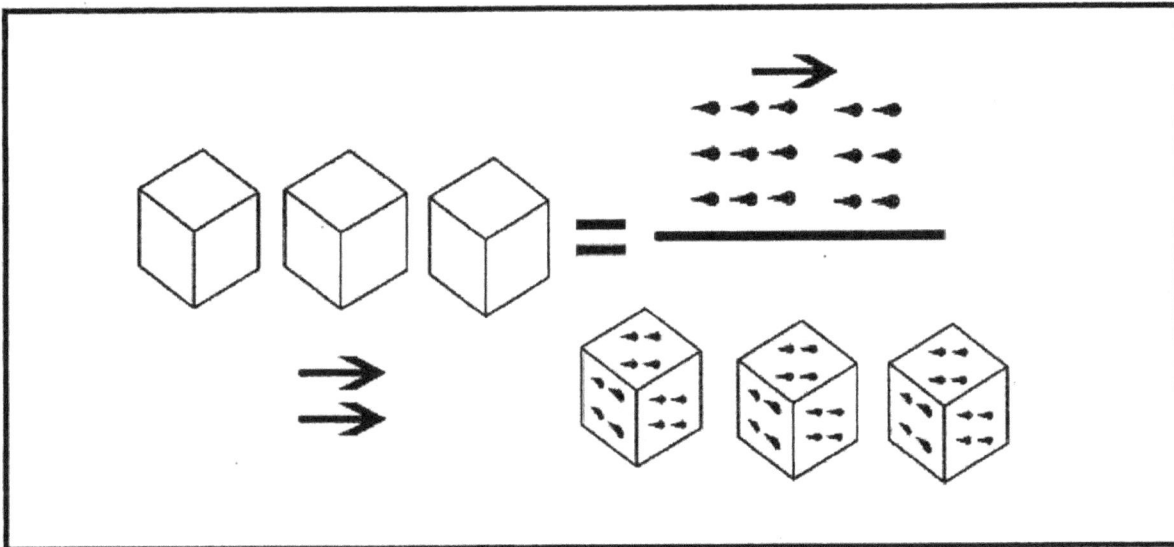

When the Flow Rate units are correct we cross multiply.

**Flow Rate = DripRate/Drop Factor**
**Flow Rate X Drop Factor = Drip Rate**

To get a physical grasp of this, the equation is saying, "the number of ml's flowing in a minute is the number of drops that fall per minute divided by the number of drops in each ml?

Let's say it in words (out loud if there's nobody around). "Flow Rate equals Drip Rate divided by Drop Factor and we want to know what the Drip Rate is".

**R E P E A T**
**5 times out loud**

Here it is in pictures. We Know (or the doctors have "given" us) the Flow Rate, the number of cc's a minute.

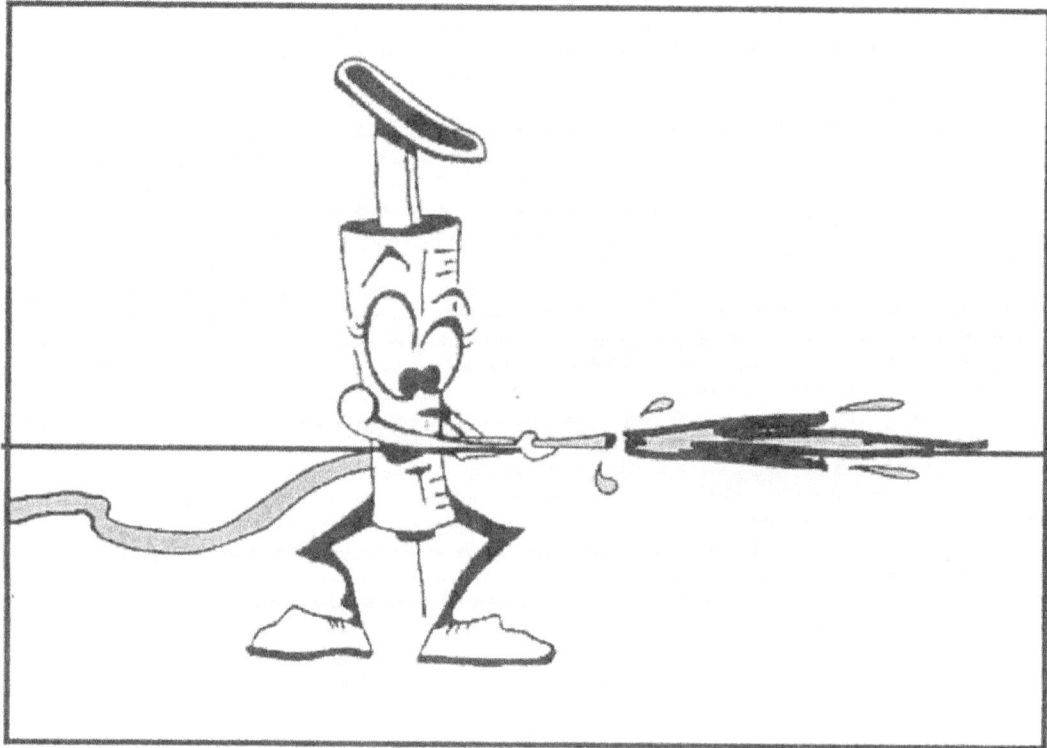

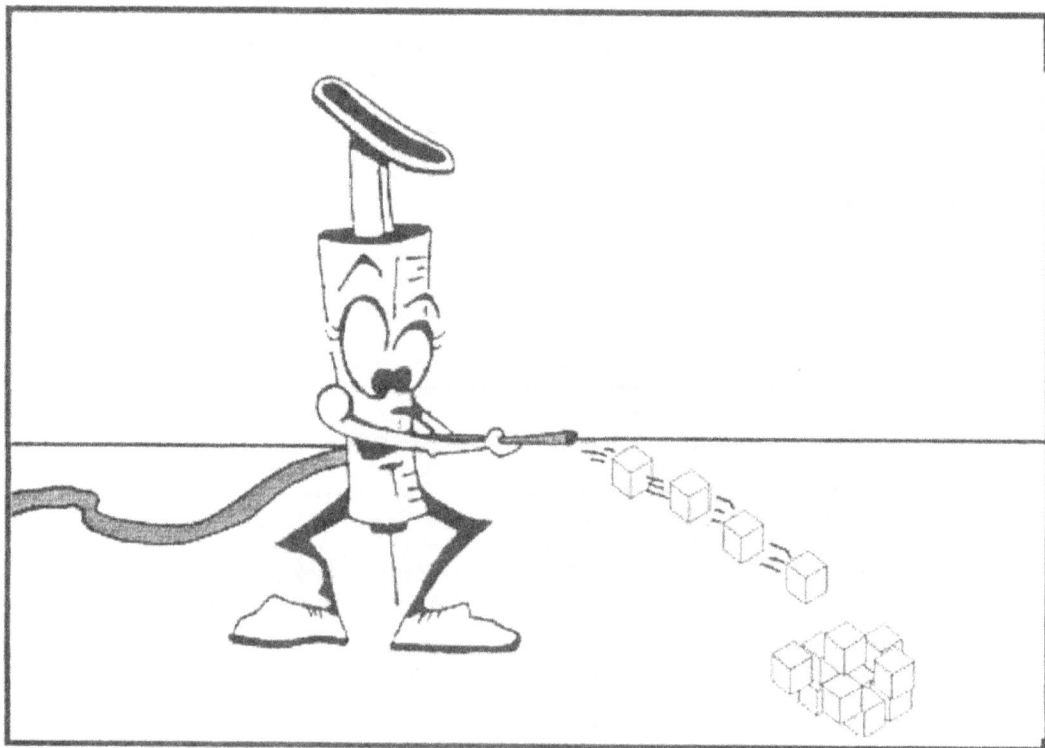

The tubing always tells us the Drop Factor - how many drops make up one cc?

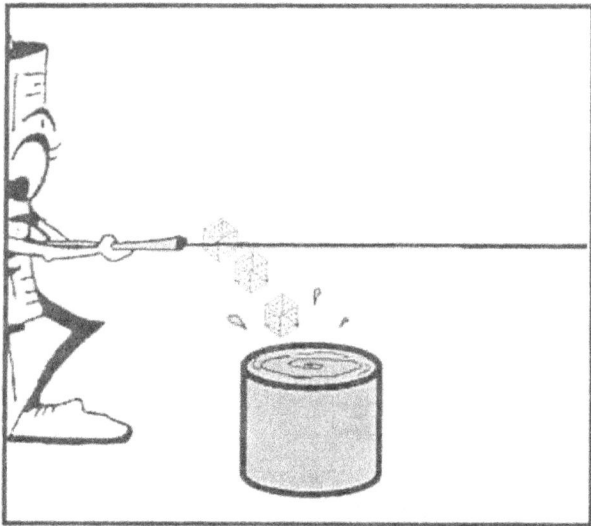

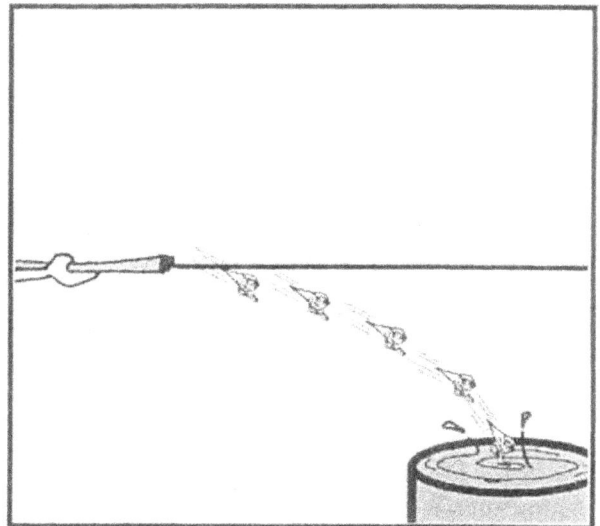

What we're being asked is how many drops (which you can count) are you going to count (in the drip chamber). What I've done is break up the total number of drops into the number of drops in each cc. And I've broken up the Flow Rate into cc's.

## W H E W ! ! ! ! !

Back to reality.
The garden hose is IV tubing and the stream is from 20cc to 125cc an hour. So the stream is more like this and if it were depicted as cc's would look like this.

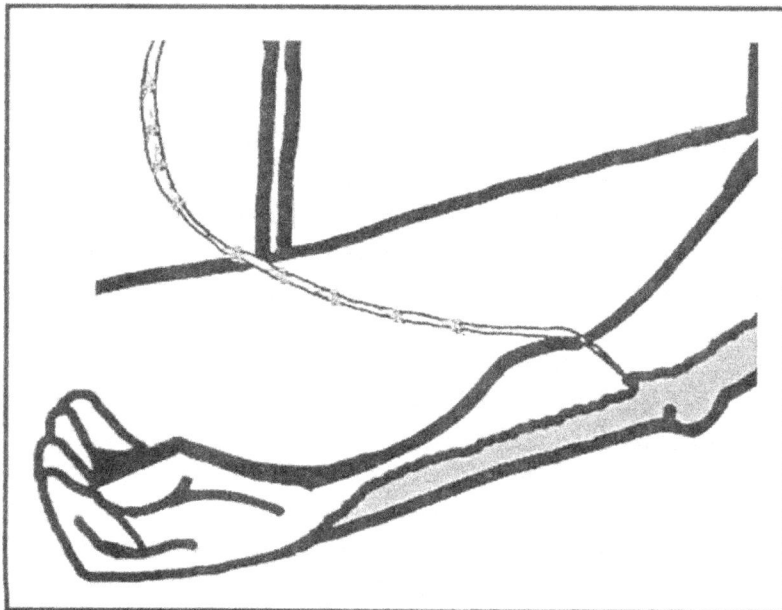

But we are doing the same thing as we did with the garden hose - counting drops and adjusting the Drip Rate into a certain (Doctor's order) Flow Rate.

## Example of Setting the Drip Rate

In this example, we are trying to set the Drop Rate at 75cc/hr. We have determined that equals 1.25 cc/min. And we know the Drop Factor is 15 gtt/cc. Now the trick is to adjust the Drip Rate with the roller clamp. On our first attempt we counted 15 gtt in a minute, that is one cc a minute, or 60cc in an hour. Too slow. We opened the roller clamp and got 20 gtt/min that's 80 cc/hr too fast. Then we slowed it to 19 gtt/min or 76 cc/hr.

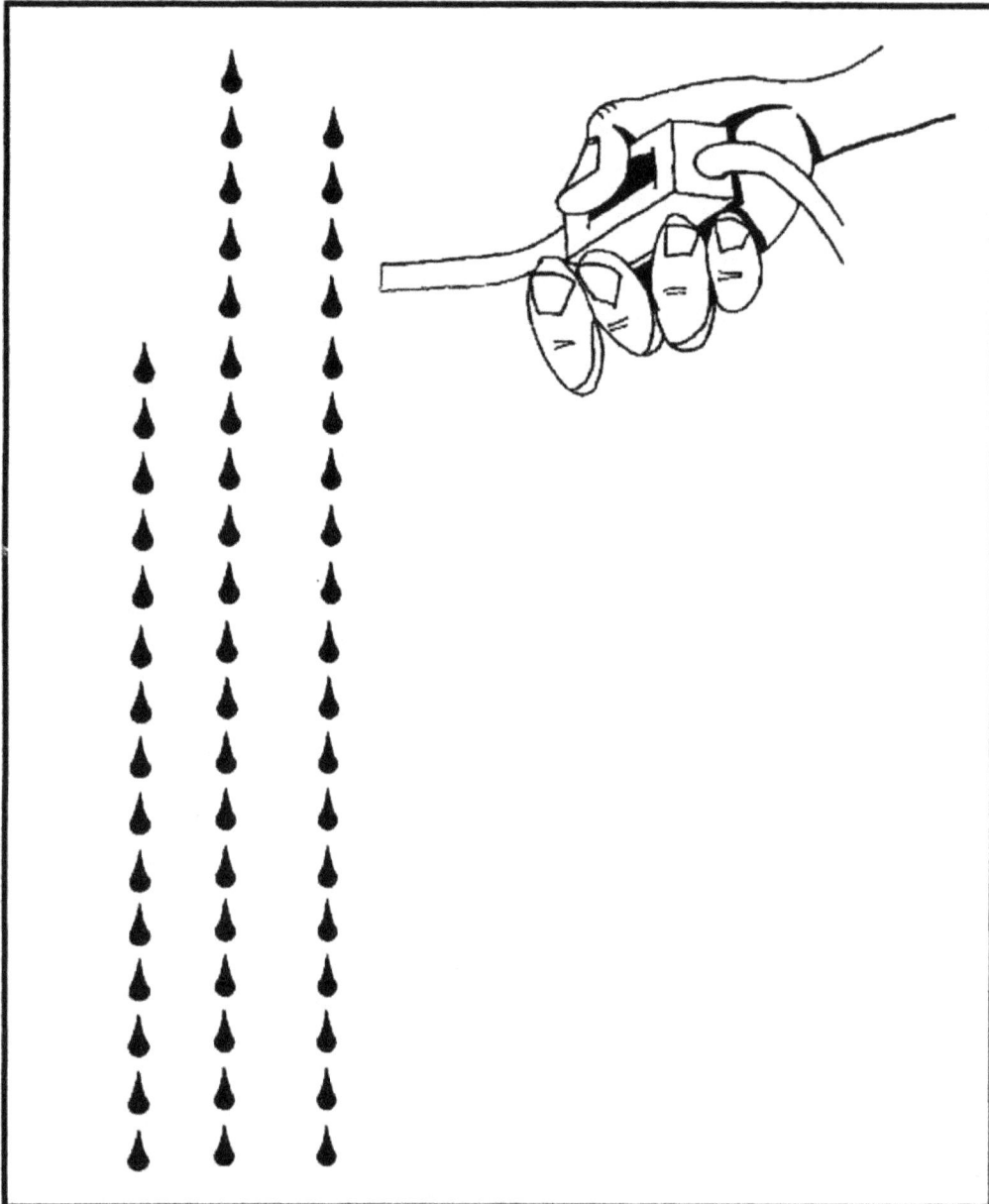

## Conclusion

You may not understand everything we've done so far. Even if you don't understand the material, glance back over the last few pages on Flow Rate, Drop Factor, Drip Rate and Conversion. Just try to see what I've tried to explain. Then go on to the following examples. I promise they will begin to make sense.

Here is a great example

The patient is in respiratory distress (can't breathe - a big problem)..
The doctor orders 200mg of aminophylline in 100cc of D5W to run for
1 hour.

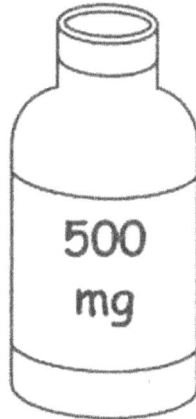

500
mg

You get a vial of aminophylline. It says 500mg in 20ml. You need 200mg.
How much do you withdraw? There is 500mg in 20ml.

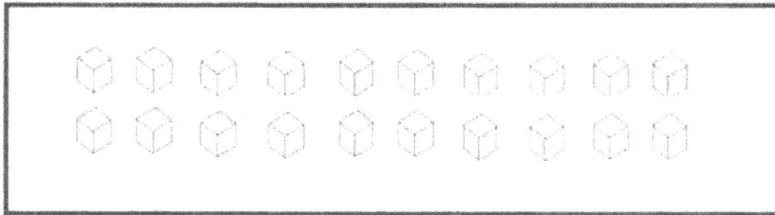

You only need 200 of those 500mg.
There are 250mg in 10ml.

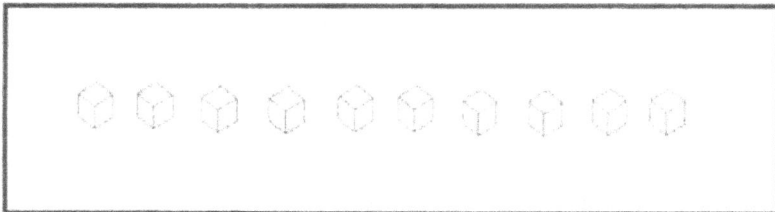

There are 25mg in each ml.

So you would withdraw 8ml for 200mg.

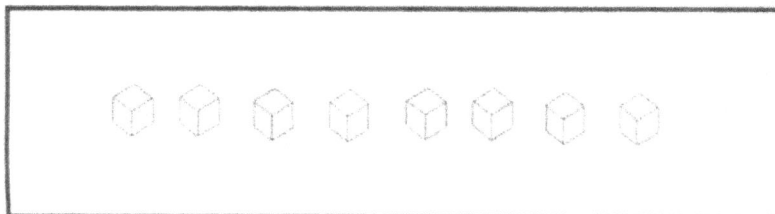

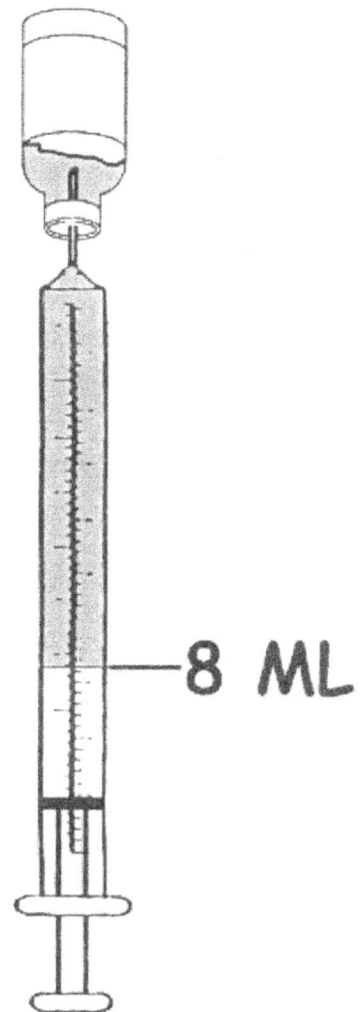

8 ML

Great Example (continued)
Then you squirt that into the 100ml bag of D5W.

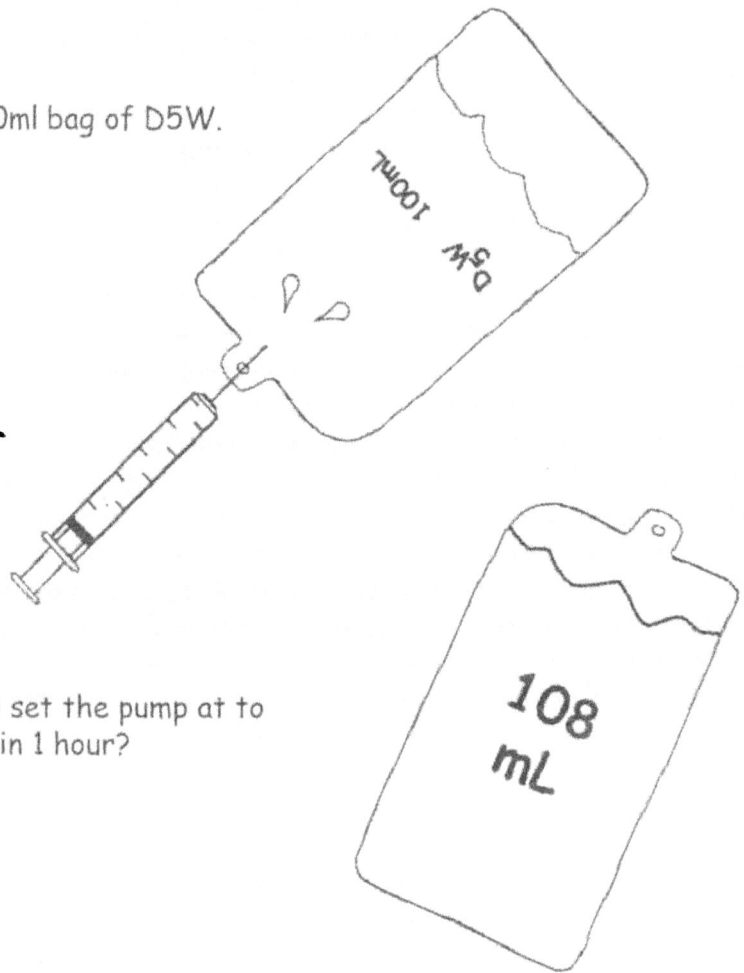

What rate do you set the pump at to run that mixture in 1 hour?

You have added 8ml to 100ml for a total of 108ml.
What rate would you set the pump at to run 108ml in 1 hour?
108ml/hour.

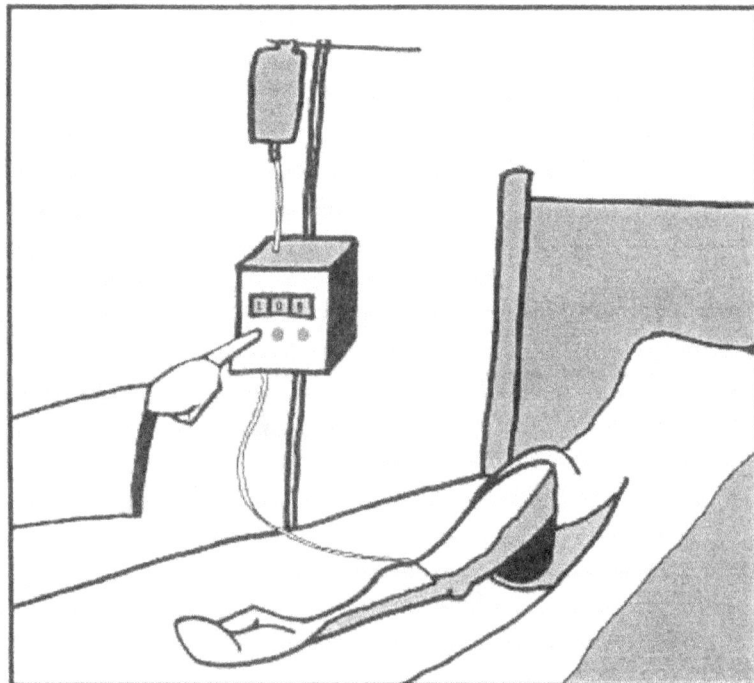

# TYPICAL DRUG TEST PROBLEMS

### (This is how they appear on drug tests- if you don't already know)

Drug ordered:          Reglan 5mg
Drug on hand:          Reglan 10mg/2ml

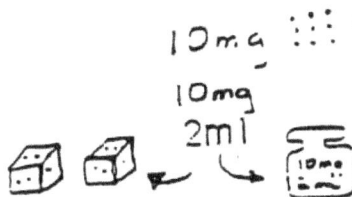

Reglan comes in a vial of 10mg/2ml.
Suppose we want 5mg.  To illustrate an intuitive approach, you would divide 2ml with 10mg by 2 to get 1ml        with 5mg.
So you would give 5mg.

Another approach would be algebra.  We know there are 10mg in 2ml and we want to know how many ml would have 5mg.  We would set this up as follows:

$$\frac{10mg}{2ml} = \frac{5mg}{xml}$$

("x" means we don't know what it is and we want to find out).

To do algebra you cross multiply, therefore $xml = \frac{5mg \times 2ml}{10mg}$

so x = 1ml.  You can use both methods.


Drug ordered:          Dilantin 25mg 1M
Drug on hand:          Dilantin 100mg/2ml

That would be very similar to the previous problem.  This one is an injection.  It comes in a 2ml vial.  We are asked how much to draw up in the syringe.

To do it intuitively, there are 100mg in 2ml.
(There **are** 100mg in there.  I just can't draw them all).  And there is 50mg in one ml.        Dividing again gives us 25mg in 1/2 ml.

Do you see how we divided until we got to 25mg? Lets try that one algebraically.

$$\frac{100mg}{2ml} = \frac{25mg}{xml}$$

Cross multiplying gives x = 1/2.  I wish I could draw in all the little milligrams to show the reality more graphically.

## Great Drip Rate Example
### (This actually happened)

The doctor wanted about 1500cc (a 1000cc bag and half a bag) to infuse in 24 hours.

While writing the order he noticed the nurse reading *Drug Calculations for Nurses Who Hate Numbers*. So... the order read, "1440cc to infuse in 24 hours or 60cc an hour or 1cc a minute or (at 15 gtt/cc) 15 gtt a minute or 1 gtt every four seconds and good luck on your math test."

1440cc
24 hours

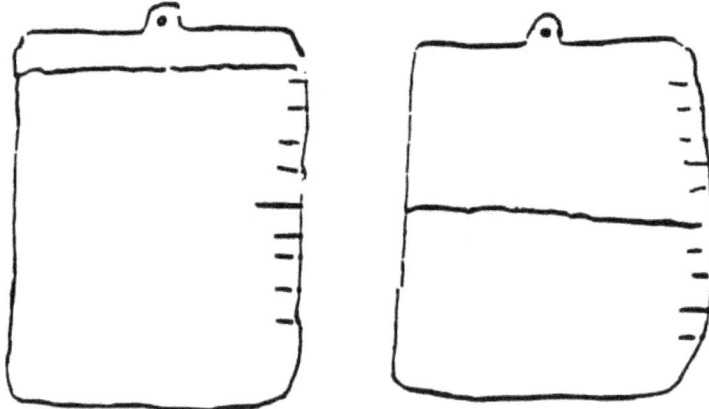

60cc
each hour

two ounces - half a cup of juice

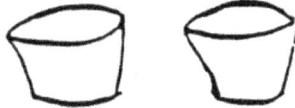

1cc
each minute

15 drops
each minute
(60 seconds)

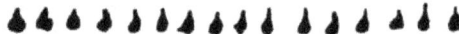

1 drop
every four
seconds

- $\dfrac{1440}{24} = \dfrac{60cc}{hour}$

  $\dfrac{60 \times 15}{60} = 15 \dfrac{gtt}{min}$

This is the easiest-to-remember method I've ever seen. Tina Hutchins, a nurse in Tennessee, showed it to me. She also helped me with many I.V. sticks.

Here it goes:

Step #1: Write down the hourly rate.
Step #2: Multiply that by the drip factor.
Step #3: Divide by 60.

I will review every problem with this method because I think you will use it on medication tests. After I saw that it worked, I tried to figure out why it worked. Let's look at a very typical example: a liter bag in 12 hours, 83cc/hr. with a 15gtt/cc drop factor.

- $$\frac{83cc}{hour} \times \frac{15gtt}{cc} \times \frac{hour}{60min} = \frac{21gtt}{min}$$

So the units work out. I always have to work out the units. It's my compulsive nature.

$$\frac{\overset{\text{Step \#1}}{83} \qquad \overset{\text{Step \#2}}{15}}{\underset{\text{Step \#3}}{60}}$$

The following pages have examples calculated by this method (they are highlighted): 56, 57, 61, and 66.

# There is nothing on this page.

( I'm not kidding. Tear the other side out and put it in your pocket)

Example #1

1000cc of D5 1/2 NS with 20mEq KCL is ordered as a continuous IV every 10 hours. The drip chamber delivers 15 drops per milliliter. How many drops per minute?

First of all what are they asking? "D5 1/2 NS with 20mEQ of KCL" is what's in the bag. For calculation of Drop Rate it doesn't matter what's in the bag. What counts is that there's a thousand cc's in one IV bag. And that it is ordered as a "continuous IV every 10 hours." That means that the doctor said it should take 10 hours for each of these bags to infuse.

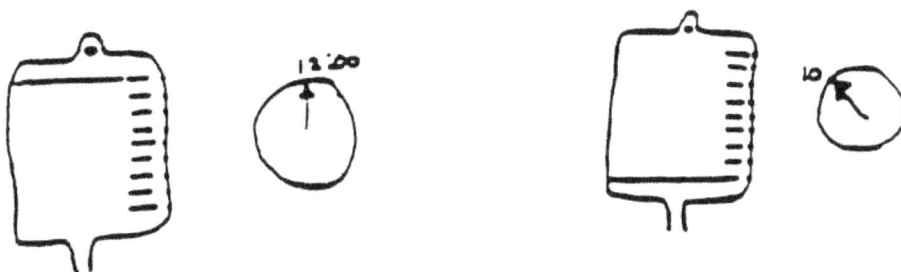

The drip chamber delivers 15 drops per millimeter or the drip chamber makes drops of a certain size. Each drop is 1/15 of a millimeter.

15 drops = 1ml

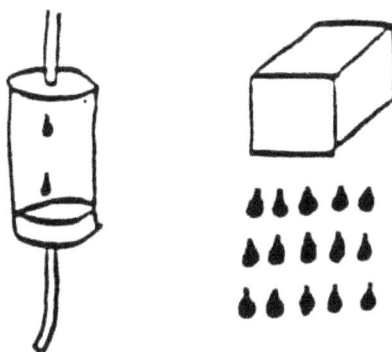

$$*\frac{1000cc}{10\ hrs} = \frac{100cc}{hour}$$

$$\frac{100\ x\ 15}{60} = \frac{25gtt}{min}$$

How many drops/minutes must flow to meet the doctor's order. Like every one of these IV questions, we are just asking what is the Flow Rate taken from the doctor's orders and put into terms which you, the nurse, can measure and give to the patient. The doctor says it should take 10 hours for this bag to flow into the patients arm and you have set the rate by adjusting the drops in the flow chamber.

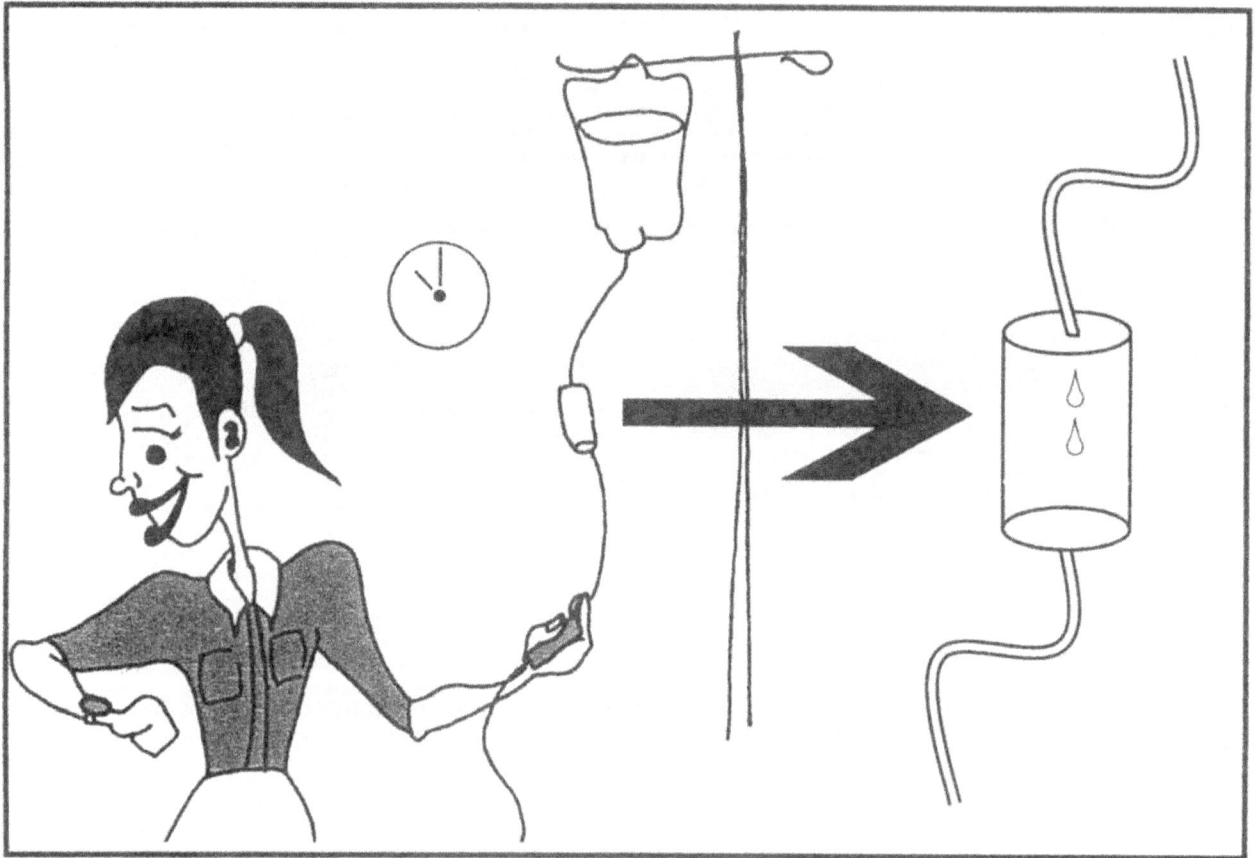

It would be very difficult to wing it and sort of aproximate how fast it should flow. It would be a lot easier to set the rate by counting the drops.

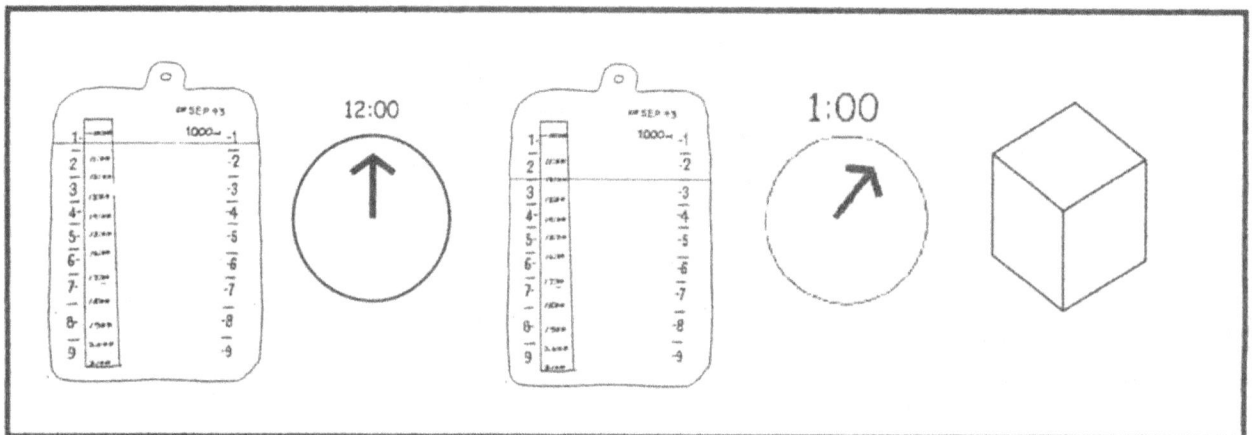

If the bag must take 10 hours then the Flow Rate is 1000cc per 10 hours or written another way 1000cc/10 hours or 100/cc per hour. But you don't have an hour to set the rate.

You need to know how much must flow in one minute (as a nurse you probably don't even have that much time). So to find out how much should flow each minute lets divide the liter bag into the total number of minutes we want it to take for the bag to finish.

We have how many minutes in 10 hours? 60 minutes in one hour and 600 minutes in 10 hours. Therefore we could rewrite the question by asking first: 1000cc must flow in 600 minutes... If 1000cc must flow in 600 minutes how many cc must flow each minute? (Remember since you're so busy you only have a minute to set the rate).

$$\frac{1000CC}{600 \ min} = \frac{1.66 \ ml}{min.}$$

Each minute is 1.66ml must flow. You could adjust the Flow Rate by getting a small measured container and a stop watch and setting the rate so it takes one minute to fill 1.66cc. Or maybe 6 minutes to fill 10ml, the same Flow Rate.

An easier way would be know how many drops equal one cc and set the Flow Rate by adjusting the drops.

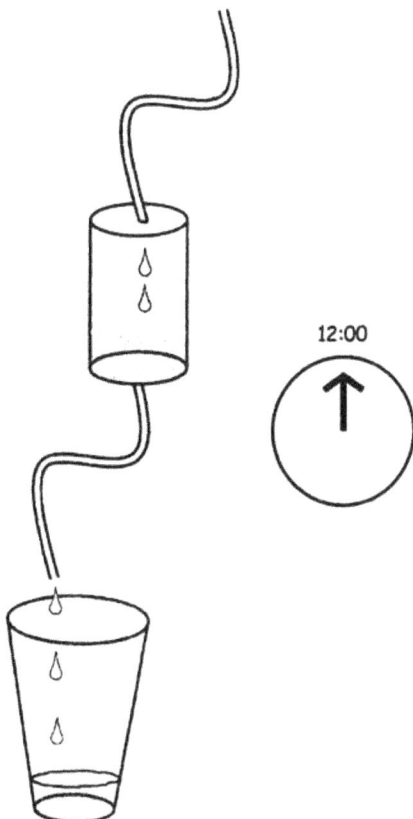

When 25 drops drip 1.66 ml will have flowed.

If 25 drops drip each minute, 1.66ml will flow each minute and in 10 hours, 1000ml will flow.

0

Here I have shown the quantities and the numbers of drops in 10 hours, one hour, and one minute.

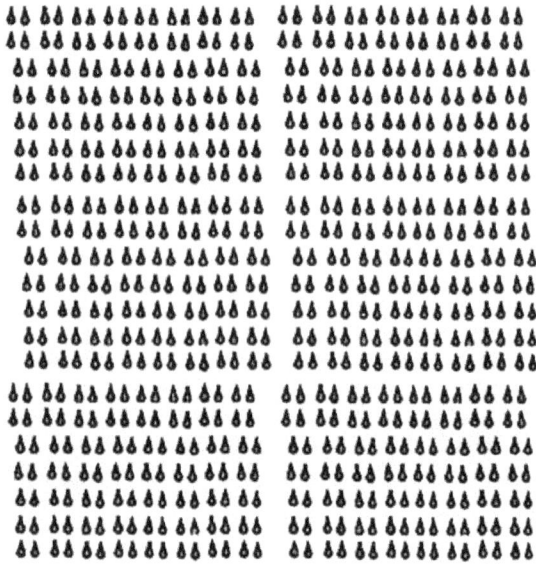

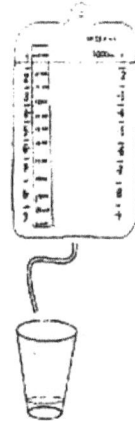

1000 cc: Approximately
1 Quart in 10 Hours
*15,000 drops*

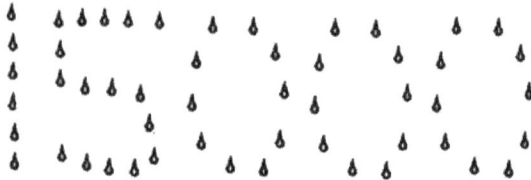

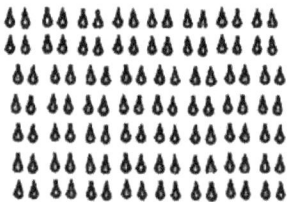

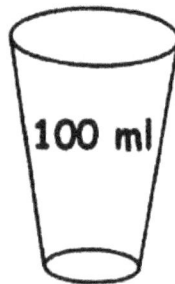

Less than a Juice Cup
Each Hour
*1,500 drops*

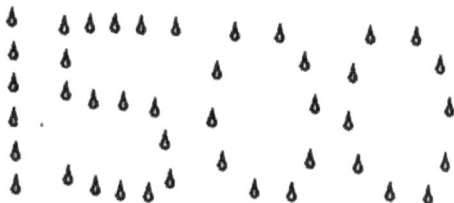

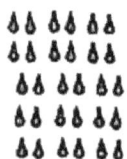

100 ml

1.66 ml
25 drops

25 drops
In one Minute.

* If I can draw 25 gtt in one minute than you should be able to count them

## Example #2

Give 500cc of 0.45 NS by IV in 10 hours.  The micro-drip set
delivers 45gtts per cc.  You will regulate the set to run at how
many drops per minute?

500 1/2 NS q10 - what the doctor meant

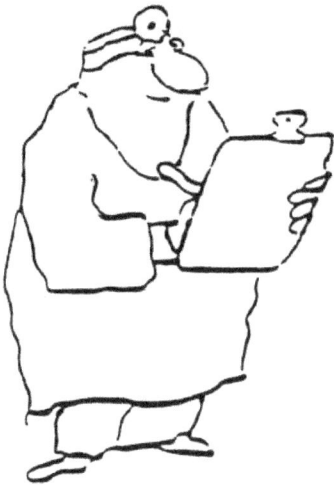

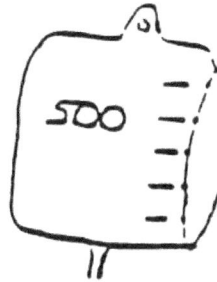

500cc 1/2 normal saline
.45 NS by IV in 10 hours.

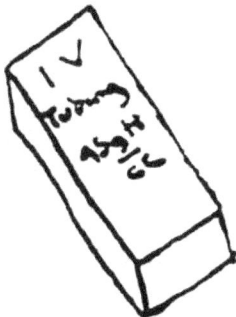

The micro-drops set delivers
45gtt per minute.

$$\frac{*500cc}{10\ hrs} = \frac{50cc}{hour}$$

$$\frac{50 \times 45}{60} = 37\ \frac{gtt}{min}$$

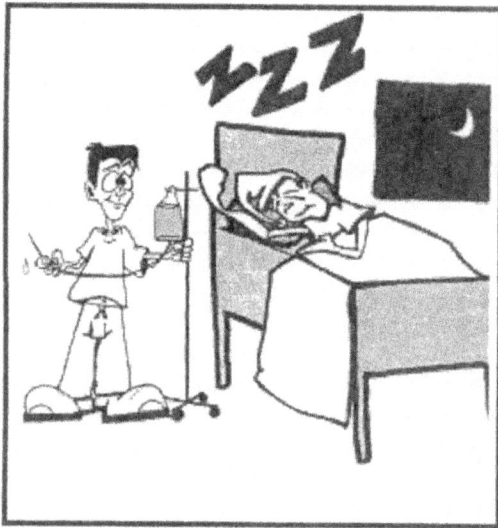

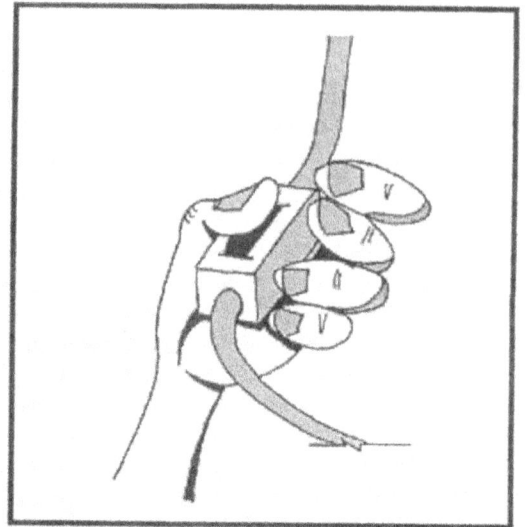

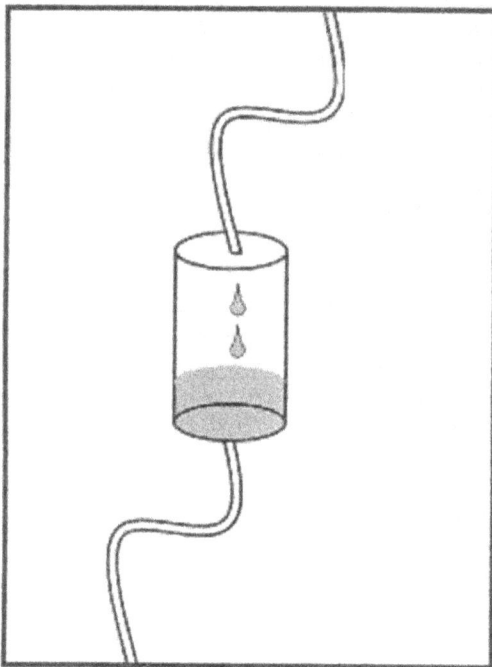

You will regulate the set to run at how many drops per minute? How many ml will the patient be receiving each hour?

What are they asking? 500ml are to flow in 10 hours.

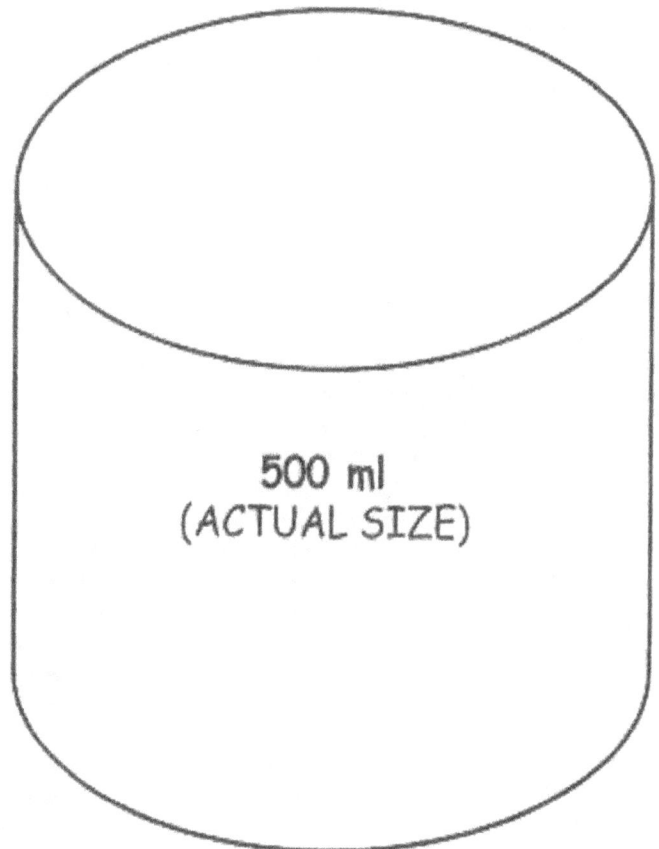

500 ml
(ACTUAL SIZE)

That's about one
pint in 10 hours...

That's 50ml in one hour.

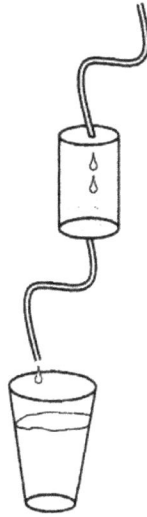

And in one minute .83ml.

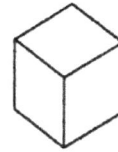

If .83ml flow in 1 minute, how many drops will drip in one minute?
There are 45gtt per ml.

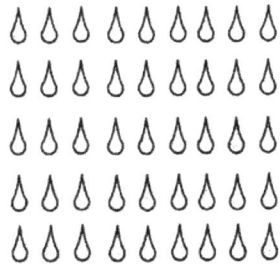 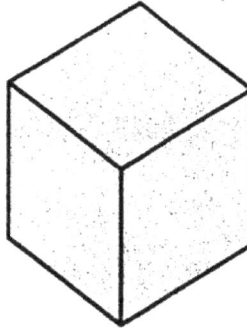 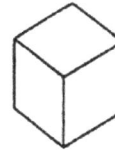

But in each minute we only get .83ml. In .83ml there are 37 of these 45 drops.

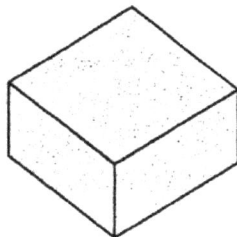 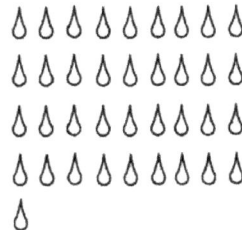 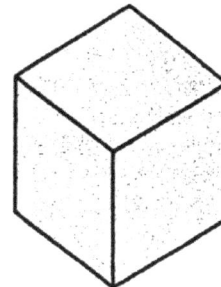

.17 ml                    .83 ml

You would adjust the Flow Rate to get 37 drops in one minute. Start out one drop every two seconds. (If one drop falls every two seconds, how many will fall in one minute? - 30 drops per minute).

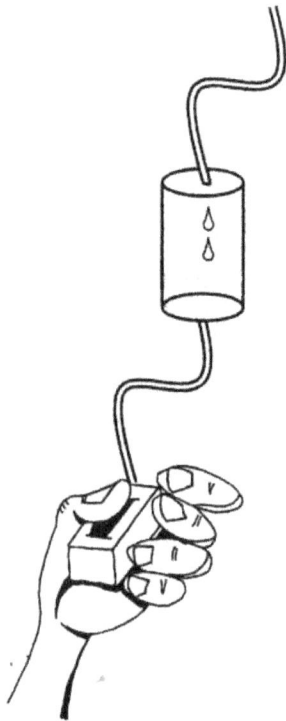

Then slow it down a little, and count for a full minute as 37 drops drip. That should bring the rate very close to 37 drops per minute.

Lets look at that problem another way using an equation. The basic format is:

$$\frac{ml}{min} = \frac{gtt/min}{gtt/ml}$$

There are always two knowns and one unknown. The question usually gives you the Flow Rate and the Drop Factor. You are usually asked to give the drip rate. That makes sense since you have no control over the doctor's order (to put it mildly). And the IV tubing you'll use is on the supply cart. So that's also a given.

What you'll be asked to do on the hospital floor is what the problem asks you to do: set the Drip Rate.

Lets look at the problem from that equation (which I asked you to memorize).

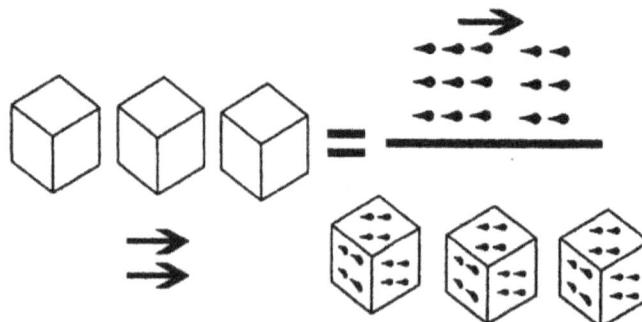

Give "500cc in 10 hours." That's the Flow Rate. First we want the Flow Rate in cc's/min.


500cc/10 hours is how many cc/min?


In 10 hours there are 600 minutes (10 hours x 60min/hour) so the Flow Rate is:

$$\frac{500cc}{600min} = .83cc/min$$

That's the Flow Rate (.83cc/minute) in the units we want to work with - cc's and minutes. Changing Flow Rate to cc/min is the only adjustment of the units you'll do.

Now we want to know how many drops per minute. We know .83cc are supposed to flow each minute and there are 45 drops in each cc, so we would multiply 45 x .83 to get 37 gtt/min.

Now lets practice setting this up real quick. Do you remember what you memorized? "Flow Rate equals Drip Rate divided by Drop Factor."

$$Flow\ Rate = \frac{?\ Drips/min}{gtt/cc} \quad (cross\ multiple\ here)$$


$$\frac{.83cc}{min} \quad x \quad \frac{45\ drops}{cc} \quad = \quad \frac{?\ drops/min}{min}$$

Canceling units and multiplying. 45 x .83 = 37, is the answer. 37gtt/min.


Once you get used to the units and you memorize the equation this should be quite routine.

Example #3

Give 500cc of 1/4 normal saline to infuse in 12 hours. The Pedi drip tubing delivers 60 gtt/cc. How many ml per hour will the patient receive? What would be the Drip Rate?

The problem says to give 500cc in 12 hours. Although you probably divided 500cc by 12 to get 41.6 or 42cc an hour. I would like to add one point here. To help visualize the Flow Rate and learn a common hospital practice with IV drips, yes put tape on the IV bag.

In the case of a drip it is important to monitor the progress for many reasons:

1. Someone on a previous shift could have set the rate incorrectly.
2. The roller valve could have loosened.

So to make sure that 42cc are flowing each hour, we often put a strip of tape on the bag to show the predicted Flow Rate against the actual time to meet the prescribed quantities.

Say you hung the 500ml bag and set the drip at 13:00, you would want to come back in an hour or so to check on the progress and you would want to leave a visible marker for the next shift to ensure the proper Flow Rate. To do this you would affix a piece of tape length-wise on the bag and mark the time pertaining to the predicted quantity.

IV bags always have quantity markers in 100cc and usually lines between showing 50cc. It looks like this:

In this case your 500cc bag which was delivering 42cc/hour would span 3 shifts. To label the tape you would figure the projected amount remaining after the first hour and mark the time, 14:00, next to the amount. 42cc have dripped and the amount left is 458. On the tape you would mark 14:00 as shown on the next page.

At 15:00 (change of shift), 500-84=416 remains. A little above 400 you would mark 15:00. For 16:00, about the time the next nurse takes over, you would be 126cc into the bag. 374cc you would mark at 16:00.

$$\frac{*500cc}{12\ hrs} = \frac{42cc}{hour}$$

$$\frac{42 \times 60}{60} = \frac{42gtt}{min}$$

The hourly marks you would make are:

14:00  -  458

15:00  -  416

16:00  -  374

17:00  -  332

18:00  -  290

19:00  -  248

20:00  -  206

21:00  -  164

22:00  -  122

23:00  -  80

24:00  -  38

And 1:00 a.m. in
the morning - done.

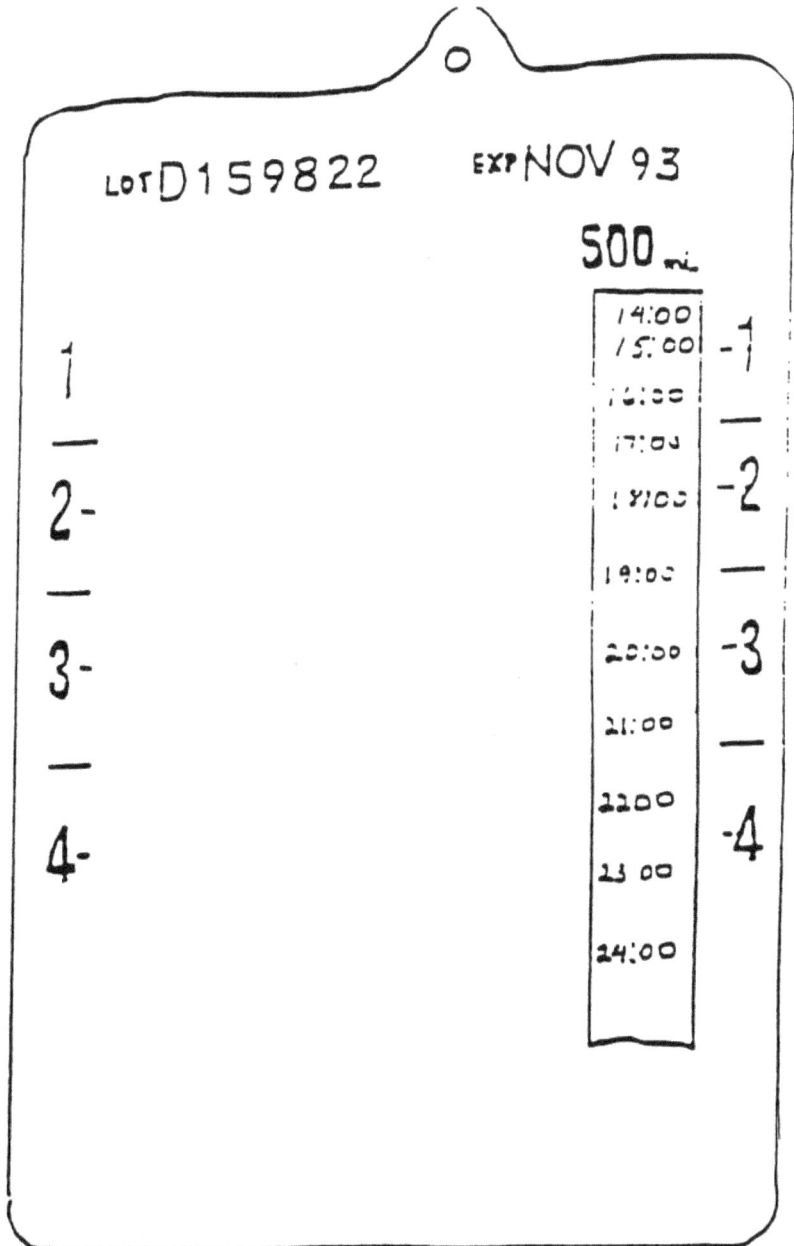

LOT D159822          EXP NOV 93

500 ml

| 14:00 | |
| 15:00 | -1 |
| 16:00 | — |
| 17:00 | |
| 18:00 | -2 |
| 19:00 | — |
| 20:00 | -3 |
| 21:00 | — |
| 22:00 | |
| 23:00 | -4 |
| 24:00 | |

1
—
2-
—
3-
—
4-

You might, or might not, have noticed that at midnight there were
38cc left.  Why not 42cc with one hour remaining?  That's because
dividing 500cc by 12 hours gives 41.66cc/hour a little less than
42, which we rounded off to.  We can do some more problems later
and I'll have some sample bags for practice.

O.K.  What's this good for?  Suppose you come on duty at 3:00,
get report, start to assess your patients and at 3:45 you notice
the bag contents at 300cc.  What does that mean?  If you look at
the tape and see that at 4:00 it should be 374cc its running a
little too fast.  You should slow the rate tightening the roller
clamp.
What rate is that?  Did I hear the word RATE?  Is that the same
rate I've been screaming and yelling about - the infamous Drip
Rate?  In fact, yes it is.  And how do you arrive at the Drip
Rate?

1. Write our equation in words, yeah "Flow Rate equals…"
2. Determine the Flow rate, 500cc in 12 hours.
3. Change the units to cc and minutes.

$$\frac{500}{12 \text{ hours}} \quad x \quad \frac{1 \text{ hour}}{60 \text{ min}} \quad = \quad \frac{.694cc}{min}$$

In 12 hours there are 720 minutes.  So the Flow Rate is 500cc/720min or .694/min.  Each minute .69cc must flow.

4. Write the equation in units.  "Flow Rate equals Drip Rate divided by Drop Factor then units:"

$$\frac{ml}{min} \quad = \quad \frac{drops/min}{drops/cc}$$

4a. (You can omit this step as you progress).  Multiply the units to show that the units cancel to give the the answer you want.

$$\frac{ml}{min} \quad = \quad \frac{drops/min}{drops/ml} \qquad \frac{ml}{min} \quad x \quad \frac{drops}{ml} \quad = \quad \frac{drops}{min}$$

I still do this.  Maybe just compulsive behavior.

5. Put in the numbers.

$$\frac{.694 \text{ ml}}{min} \quad = \quad \frac{? \text{ drops/min}}{60 \text{ drops/ml}}$$

$$\frac{.694 \text{ ml}}{min} \quad x \quad \frac{60 \text{ drops}}{ml} \quad = \quad 41.64 \quad = \quad \frac{42 \text{ drops}}{min} \text{(close enough)}$$

# Example #4

Determine the Drip Rate of an IV infusion so if the doctor ordered 1000ml to be given in 3.6 hours the tubing delivers 10 gtt/ml.

1.) Identify the information that's given. The Flow Rate is 1000ml in 3.6 hours, 1000ml/3.6 Hours. The Drop Factor is 10gtt/ml.

2.) Change the units to ml/min. There are 216 min in 3.6 hours. The Flow Rate in ml/min is 1000ml/216 min or 4.63 ml/min.

3.) Write the equation in words Flow Rate = Drop Rate divided by Drop Factor.

4.) Then units

$$\frac{ml}{min} = \frac{Drop/min}{Drop/ml}$$

5.) Check to make sure these units work correctly

$$\frac{ml}{min} = \frac{Drops/min}{Drops/ml} \qquad \text{Cross Multiply} \qquad \frac{ml}{min} \times \frac{Drops}{ml} = \frac{Drops}{min}$$

### The Units Checks Out

Put the numbers in

$$\frac{4.63\ ml}{min} = \frac{?\ Drops/min}{10\ Drops/ml}$$

46.3= 46 Drops/min (as close as you'll get)

## Example #5

Let's try a situation that leaves some judgement to you.  The order says 500mg Primaxin IV, that's all.  You look at the patients medicine drawer and see a vial of Primaxin R, which is a white powder.

You have to dilute it and set the rate.  The doctor did not say how.  He's trusting you to do it correctly.  First look up what to dilute it in.  The top of the vial says dilute it in "Normal Saline."

10cc normal saline vials are all over the place.  Take the normal saline, inject it into the vial of Primaxin R, shake it.  See if it dissolves into clear liquid.  Go to the supply cart.  Get a small bag, say 250cc of normal saline, and tubing with a Buritrol.  Hang the bag, fill the Buritrol with - how much?  We look on the dilution chart and see 500mg of Primaxin should be diluted in 100cc of normal saline.  So fill the Buritrol with 100cc then withdraw the Primaxin liquid from the vial and inject it into the Buritrol.  Flush the patient's Hep Lock with 2cc of normal saline and connect the tubing to the Hep Lock.  Then set the Drip Rate.  Sorry about that.  Back to the numbers.

In general a normal adult could receive 100cc in an hour.  That's a little less than a 4 oz. juice container, so setting the drip rate for 100cc/hour would be safe.  It would not over hydrate most people.

100cc/hour is how many drops per minute.  We look at the tubing to find the Drop Factor; it is always there.  Say it says 15 drops per cc.  First write the equation:

$$\text{Flow Rate} = \frac{\text{Drip Rate}}{\text{Drop Factor}}$$

We know the Drop Factor and we know the Flow Rate, except not in the right units.

$$\frac{100cc}{Hour} = \frac{?\ \text{Drip Rate}}{15\ \text{Drops/cc}}$$

Change the Flow Rate to minutes and put it in the equation. 100cc in one hour is 100cc in 60 minutes or 100cc/60min = 1.66cc/min:

Another way: $\dfrac{1.66cc}{min} = \dfrac{?\ gtt/min}{15gtt/cc}$

$\dfrac{1.66cc}{min} \times \dfrac{15gtt}{cc} = 24.99\ gtt/min = 25\ gtt/min$

You would start by adjusting the rate to one drop every 2 seconds or 30 gtt.  Then slow it down a little, then get to about 6 drops in 15 seconds and you have it.

## Example #6

*Setting a Pump Rate*

The doctor's orders might say "2000 liters in 24 hours," or they might say "one liter to finish at 8 p.m." and you would have to read a little into this.  Knowing that the doctor had made rounds this morning, you would understand the meaning was a twelve hour running time.  If you did not see the order until 8:45 and did not hand the bag until 9:15, you would figure a finishing time of 12 hours later, 9:15 p.m. or 21:15.  If you had a volumetric IV pump you would set it at 83cc/hour.  Another typical order is 1000cc in 12 hours – also 83cc/hour.

To get a feel for the true quantities involved, try turning on your kitchen sink at a rate where it would fill a little more than 2 1/2 ounces in an hour.  That would be what you're setting the pump at – that's a very small flow for your faucet but a very typical IV Flow Rate.

## Example #7

The physician orders "2 mg per minute of Lidocaine Stat." Using 500 ml of D5W and 2gms of Lidocaine, how many cc's per minute will you administer?

In this case the doctor wants to inject the Lidocaine intravenously. But to avoid a reaction it must be diluted. So the 2gms are diluted in a 500ml bag.

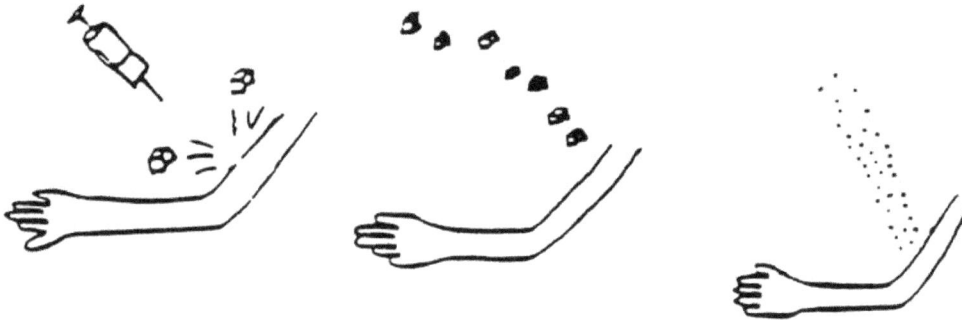

You would first go to the Med Room and get a 500cc bag of D5W. Then you would look in the cabinet for Lidocaine R.

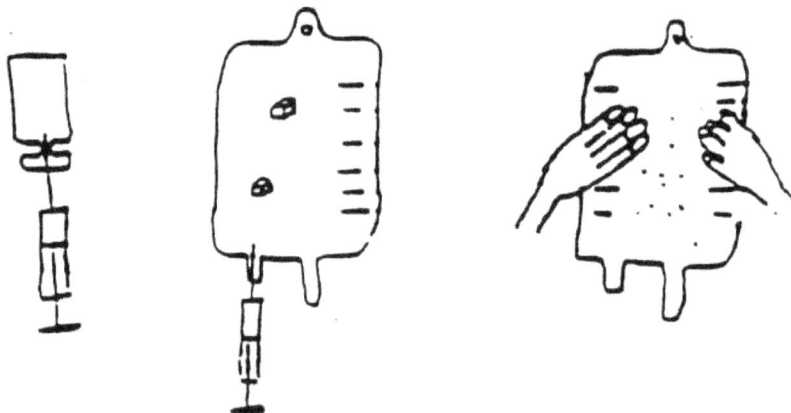

The 2gms of Lidocaine R would come in a small vial about 10ml. They would be drawn from the vial by syringe and injected into the 500ml bag and mixed. Now we have 2gms or mixed in 500cc (500 + 10).

You will remember that a paper clip weighs about 1gm and that a milligram is 1/1000 of a gram.

So instead of seeing 2gms injected into 500cc, we could see 2000 milligrams.

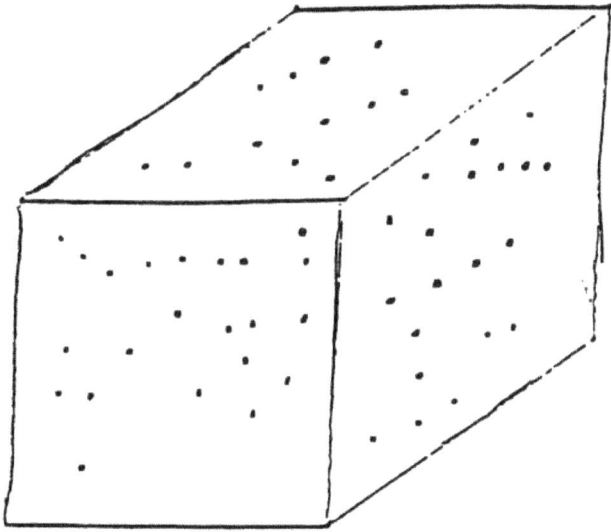

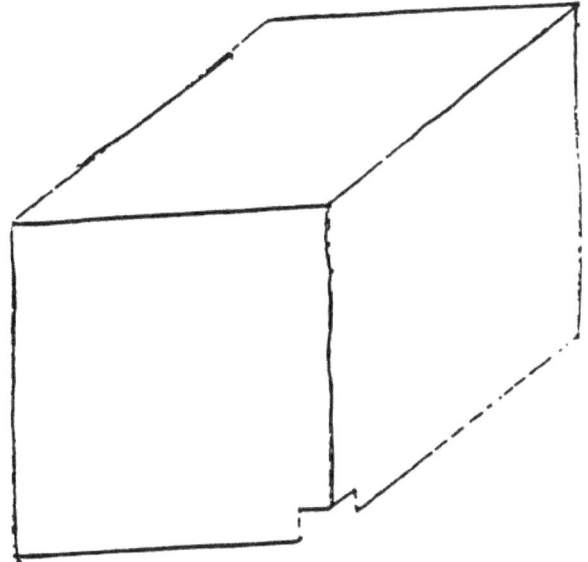

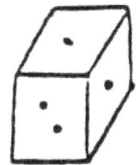

How many milligrams would be in each of the 500cc's?  How many milligrams are in each cc if there are 2000 milligrams in 500cc?

In each cc there would be 2000 milligrams/500cc:

$$\frac{2000mg}{500cc} = \frac{4 \text{ milligrams}}{cc}$$

4 milligrams/cc in each of the 500cc.  If the doctor wants 2mg
per minute and you know there are 4mg/ml, how many ml/min would
you infuse?

There are 4mg in each cc of fluid.  But we only need 2.  So 1/2ml
of fluid would have 2mg.

If 1/2 cc flow each minute
30cc will flow each hour.

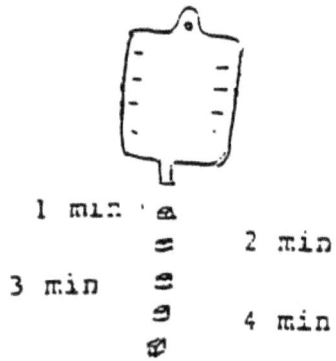

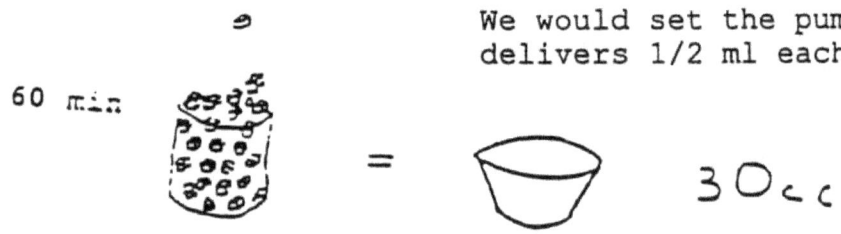

1 min    2 min

3 min

4 min

60 min

We would set the pump at a rate that
delivers 1/2 ml each minute or 30cc/hr.

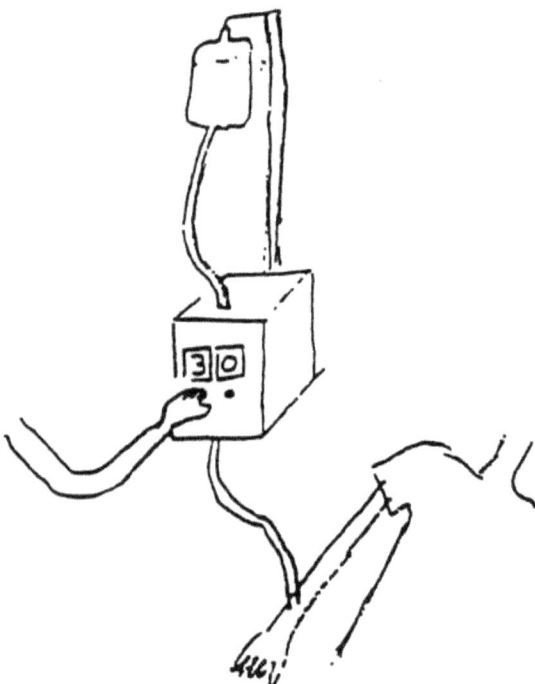

= 30cc

# Example #8

Here's a true to life example. In the report they told me "**Lido Drip at two mg a minute**". To look intelligent, I said "o.k.". When I walked in the room to check, I saw the following:

1.) The bag of Lidocaine labeled 2g in 250ml of D5W
2.) The pump was running at 15cc/hr.

Hmmmmmm... Lets see if that jives...
2 Grams in 250ml. That's 2000mg in 250ml or 2000mg/250ml = 8mg/ml
15ml/hr and 8mg in each ml is 120mg an hour.

But that's in one hour. To find out how many mg flow in one minute we would divide the number of mg that flow in an hour (120mg) by 60 to get ... 2mg/min: Or 15ml/hour divided by 60 gives us 1/4ml/min. Since there were 8mg in each ml there are 2mg in 1/4ml.

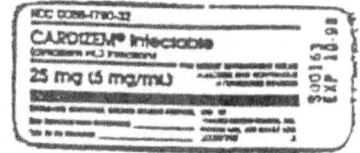

## Example #9

When I call the pharmacy to ask about a rate, there is usually a problem (example) for this book.  So here it goes: The patient's heart rate was about 150.  I called the cardiologist.  He said, "Put him on a cardizem drip.  Titrate to keep the rate below 110."  I said (because I had no idea what to do), "Where do I start?"  He said, "5mg an hour to a max of 30mg an hour."  I wrote it on the orders and called the pharmacy.

They told me what do to.  Put 125mg in 100ml of D5W.  The three vials of cardizem contained 5mg/ml, two 10ml vials and one 5ml.  So 125mg of cardizem was 25ml.  Adding 25ml of cardizem to 100ml of D5W equals 125ml.  That's one mg in each ml.

So 5mg an hour is 5ml an hour on the pump.  His heart rate didn't drop much.  So I increased the rate to 7ml/hour.  Which is how many mg/hr?  7.  Right?

| DILUTION | | ADMINISTRATION | |
|---|---|---|---|
| Diluent Volume | Quantity of Cardizem Injection | Dose | Infusion Rate |
| 100 mL | 125 mg (25 mL) | 5 mg/hr | 5 mL/hr |
| | | 10 mg/hr | 10 mL/hr |
| | | 15 mg/hr | 15 mL/hr |
| 250 mL | 250 mg (50 mL) | 5 mg/hr | 6 mL/hr |
| | | 10 mg/hr | 12 mL/hr |
| | | 15 mg/hr | 18 mL/hr |
| 500 mL | 250 mg (50 mL) | 5 mg/hr | 11 mL/hr |
| | | 10 mg/hr | 22 mL/hr |
| | | 15 mg/hr | 33 mL/hr |

5 mg/hr ≈ 180 mg/day oral steady state*
7 mg/hr ≈ 240 mg/day oral steady state*
11 mg/hr ≈ 360 mg/day oral steady state*

*Based on pharmacokinetic studies in normal subjects

## CONVENIENT DOSAGE

**1** Beginning treatment as

**BOLUS:** 0.25 mg/kg actual body weight over 2 minutes

20 mg average patient

**2** If response is inadequate, wait 15 minutes

**BOLUS:** 0.35 mg/kg actual body weight over 2 minutes

25 mg average patient

**3** Treatment as

**INFUSION:** 10 to 15 mg/hr in some patients a 5 mg/hr starting infusion may be appropriate

## CARDIZEM INJECTABLE . . . CONTROL* THAT IS FAST, SAFE, AND CONTINUOUS

*Conversion to normal sinus rhythm no greater than placebo.

Please see enclosed prescribing information.

## Example #9

We're going to turn up the rate here... the rate of IV knowledge intake.

In this problem we'll look at a Heparin Drip. Heparin is a blood thinner. It usually appears in the doctor's order when people's blood clots. That makes sense. Right? Doctor's adjust the rate by blood coagulation test. Quantities of Heparin are given in "units". A typical order would look like this:

Translated into legible english letters that means "25000 units of Herparin in 500cc of D5w @ 900 units/hour". Although we might call this a Herparin Drip, Herparin would always be on a pump. What we need to do is set the pump rate. First lets look at 25000 units in 500cc.

How many are in each cc?

$$\frac{25000 \text{ Units}}{500\text{cc}}$$

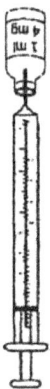

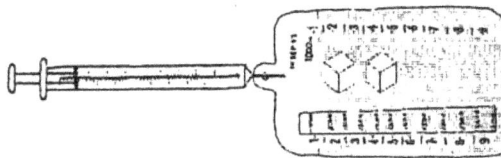

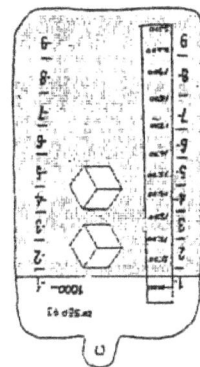

50 Units

There are 50 units in each cc the doctor wants 900 units an hour. If there are 50/units in each cc, how many cc would give us 900 units?

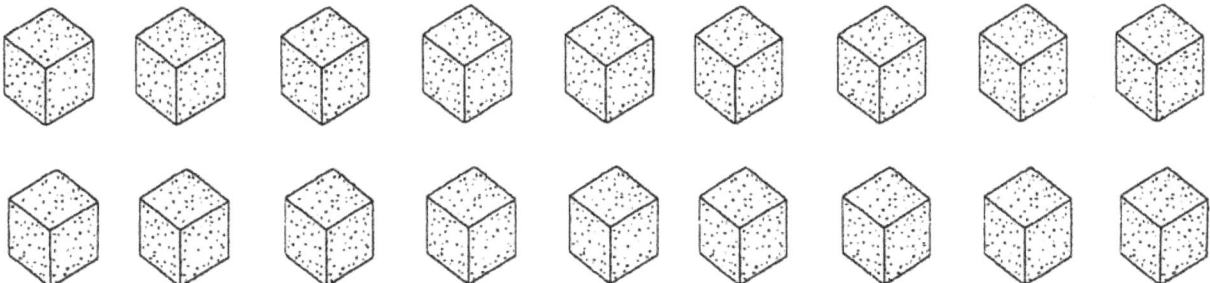

18cc's give us 900 units <u>500 units/cc</u>. We would need that many an hour. We would set the pump at 18cc per hour.

# One Final Thought

In my LPN_RN transition course there were IV problems. The bad part was that after having written a book on the subject, I still had to repeat the whole thought process each time.

Since you now understand the IV Flow Rates, here is a memory device to quickly set up the problems.

Do you see how the Flow Rate in cc's equals the Flow Rate in drops if we divide by the number of drops in each cc.

Just put the given information into the picture.

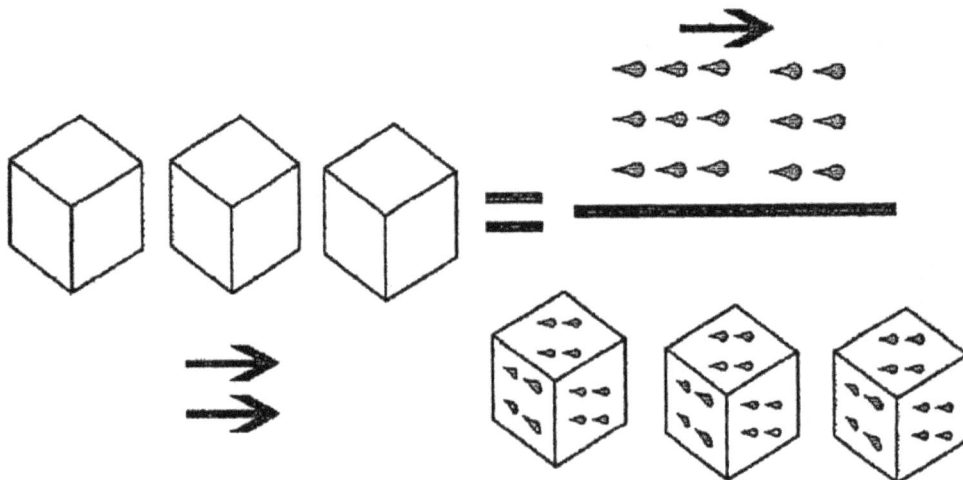

*This picture will never let you down.*

# PITOCIN

"Pitocin 10 units in 500cc D5W @ 6 millilunits/min"

For drug calculations pitocin is great. It comes in units and milliunits. When "milli" precedes an amount it means 1/1000 of that amount. Milligram means 1/1000 of a liter. Milliunit means 1/1000 of a unit.

Pitocin is administrated by I.V. infusion to augment contractions in labor and delivery. Increasing the infusion rate increases the strength and frequency of contractions. The rate starts low, usually at about 6 milliunits/min.

Our problem is to set the pump in milliliters/hour (ml/hr) when the orders are in milliunits/min and the I.V. bag is units of pitocin mixed in D5W. What we are going to do is set the pump rate (cc/hr) so the infusion delivers the right amount of pitocin (milliunits/min) from an I.V. bag (units mixed in 500ml of solution).

Lets say the ordered infusion rate is 6 milliunits/min. The solution in the bag is 10 units of pitocin added to 500cc D5W.

First lets look at the bag. If there are 10 units of pitocin in 500cc D5W, there are also 10,000 milliunits. That's because a unit is composed of 1000 milliunits. How many milliunits are in each cc of solution?

$$\frac{10,000 \text{ milliunits}}{500cc} = \frac{20 \text{ milliunits}}{cc}$$

There are 20 milliunits in each cc.
We need 6 milliunits each minute.
How many cc/hr of solution do we need to provide 6 milliunits each minute?

To do this first convert milliunits/min to milliunits/hr. Since there are 60 minutes in an hour, we multiply the desired 6 milliunits/min by 60 to get 360 milliunits/hr.
We want 360 milliunits each hour and we know that there are 20 milliunits in each cc.
Since there are twenty milliunits in each cc
We need 18 cc to give us 360 milliunits
By setting the pump at 18cc/hr we can get 360 milliunits/hr or 6 milliunits/min.

# Ask Your Pharmacist How To Do This One

Tylenol #3 contains 300mg of acetaminophen and 30mg of codiene (which is why it is a narcotic). Tylenol #2 contains 300mg of acetaminophen and 15mg of codeine.

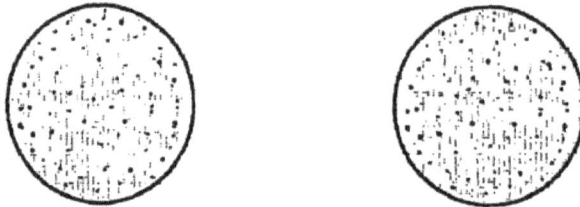

The doctor orders Tylenol #2. Your hospital only carries Tylenol #3. What can you do?

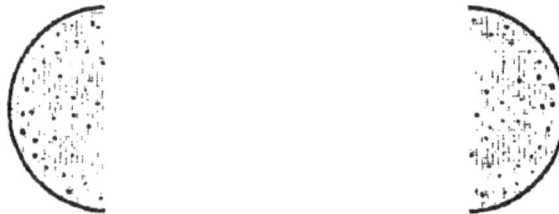

Obviously the codiene is a stronger consideration than the acetaminophen. So you would begin by splitting the Tylenol #3 in two. That would give you 15mg of codeine and 150mg of acetaminophen. To get the other 150mg of acetaminophen, split a regular Tylenol tablet (325mg) in half. That would give you 162mg - which is probably close enough. 150+162=312mg acetaminophen and 15mg of codeine.

## Example #11

Solumedrol comes in a vial with 40mg in 1ml. You want 15mg. You could use algebra :

$$\frac{x \text{ ml}}{15mg} = \frac{1 \text{ ml}}{40mg} \quad x \text{ ml} \quad \frac{15mg}{40mg} \qquad x=.375$$

I like another way: each 5mg is 1/8 of 4mg. So 15mg is 3/8 of 40mg. 3/8 of a ml.

## Example #12

Here is a problem that tests your eyesight. The doctor orders 12.5 grams of Manitol. Manitol is a very strong diuretic. The 50ml vial says in very small print, 250 milligrams in each ml.

In each vial of 50ml there are 250mg, so there are a total of 50 (number of milliliters) x 250 (number of milligrams) of Maintol in each ml. 50 x 250 = 12,500. So 12,500mg is 12.5 grams.

## Example #13

"Phoslo 2001mg PO AC Meals"

That's a pretty weird order. 2000mg isn't enough? An extra mg for good measure. A 2001mg tablet? Yeah right. "Hey everyone, get a load of this."

It turns out to make sense. Tablets are 667mg, so

667 + 667 + 667 = 2001

Do you believe it?

```
PHOSLO
CALCIUM
ACETATE
667MG TAB
EXP: 09/30/98
LOT: UP71249900
```

Example #14
"Levothyroxine 25mcg I.V."

Levothyroxine, sythroid, I.V. comes in a vial of 200mcg (micrograms) of powder. The instructions say reconstitute with 5ml sterile water - which you do, no problem. You now have 200 micrograms in your vial.

You need 25 micrograms. How much do you withdraw? I would do it as follows: 25mcg is 1/8 of 200mcg. Therefore, you want 1/8 of 5ml. 1/8 of 5ml is .625ml. A 1ml tubercular syringe would be perfect.

Example #15

The patient was on synthoid 0.100mg P.O. Q.D. She had already gotten the pill when the doctor increased the dose to 0.125mg Q.D. The pharmacy sent 0.125. I didn't know what to do. I called the pharmacy and asked for a 0.025mg pill. The pharmacist suggested that I take a 0.100mg pill, which was already in the patient's med drawer and split it into 4 pieces for the extra 0.025mg. I knew that.

Example #16
Concentration

Aminophylline 500mg in 250cc 1/2 N.S. @ 10cc/hr.

Concentration - that is always a potential for mistakes. I picked up a COPP patient in the Emergency room. The order read 500mg of Aminophylline in 250cc 1/2 N.S. at 10cc/hour. Apparently on nights they didn't have 250cc bags of 1/2 N.S. So they put 500mg of Aminophylline in 500cc of 1/2 N.S. and ran it at 20cc. That comes out to the same Aminophylline infusion rate of 20mg/hour. But I immediately changed the bag to the ordered concentration. It looked like a mistake waiting to happen. I could imagine the correct bag coming from pharmacy and the pump staying at 20cc/hour. And it brings up the importance of checking the concentration - especially if you are using charts. One last comment concerning the concentration. I think it would have been more prudent to mix 250mg of aminophylline in 250cc of 1/2 N.S. That way the pump could have been set at the prescribed rate and when the correct mix came there would be no change.

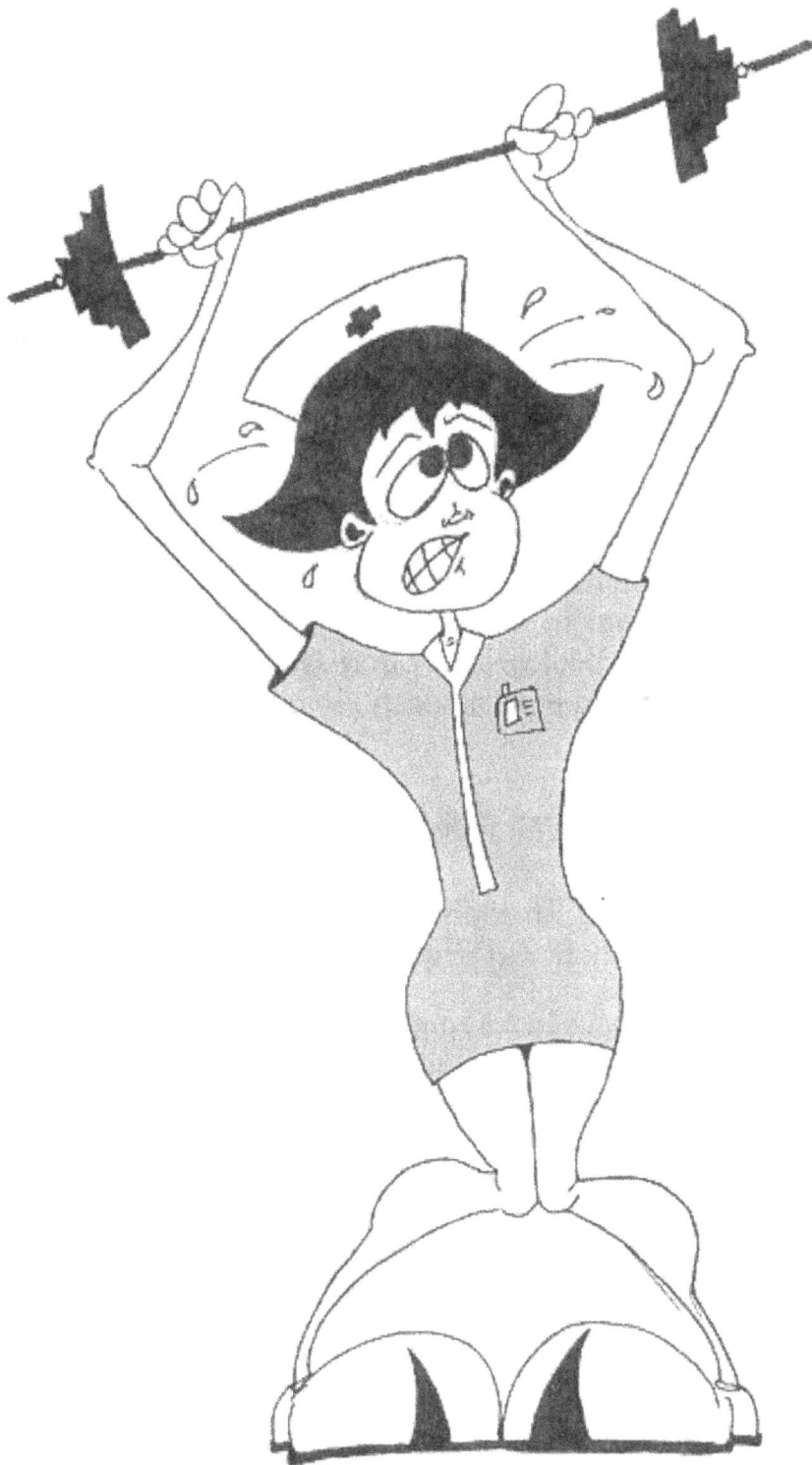

WEIGHTS

# CONVERTING POUNDS TO KILOGRAMS

In school and in real nursing situations, you will frequently need to convert pounds and ounces to kilograms and milligrams.

A pound you probably know intuitvely. A pint of water weighs about a pound. A way to remember that is "A pint is a pound the whole world round." There is a volume ounce and a weight ounce. A volume ounce of water weighs about an ounce - which I think is the reason they are both called an ounce. A pill cup is approximately a volume ounce. Full of water it weighs about an ounce. 16 pill cups, or 16 volume ounces equal a pint. 16 pill cups full of water weigh about a pound.

A kilogram equals 2.2 pounds. There are two ways to remember this: #1 You would rather weigh yourself in kilograms than pounds. The number of kilograms you weigh will always be less than half the number of pounds you weigh. Since there are 2.2 lbs in each kilogram, your weight in kilograms is your weight in pounds divided by 2.2. #2 A liter of water weighs a kilogram. A liter is about the same as a quart. A quart is two pints which are about a pound each. So a liter weighs a little more than two pounds - 2.2 to be exact.

## Ounces and Milligrams

In each pound there 16 ounces. In each kilogram are 1000 milligrams. A liter of water weighs a kilogram. A milliliter of water weighs a milligram.

Lets try a conversion from ounces to milligrams. Do you remember the pill cup full of water. It weighs an ounce. At the full line you'll see 30ml. To be exact 31 milligrams equals an ounce. By this example of conversion, there are 31mg in an ounce (weight) since there are about 30ml in an ounce (volume) of water.

Lets try some more examples : 16lbs is how many kilograms. Remember you weigh less in kilograms. So divide by 2.2.   16/2.2=5kg
66lb is how many kg?  66/2.2=30kg.

Let's try some conversions that are a little harder.
8 lbs. 2 oz. is how many mg?

8 lbs./2.2 = 3.63kg or 3630mg.

Each ounce is 31mg.   2 oz. = 62 mg.

Therefore, 8 lbs. 2 oz. = 3630 mg + 62 mg = 3692 mg or 3.69 kg.


A 6 ½ pound baby girl weighs how many kg?  Since there are 16 ounces in a pound, 6 ½ lbs. is 6 lbs. 8 oz.

6/2.2 = 2.72 kg = 2720 mg.

8 oz. x 31 = 248 mg.    2720 mg + 248 mg = 2968 mg.

2968 mg is 2.97 kg (rounding off).

Or you could have divided 6.5 lbs. by 2.2 to get 2.95 kg.  The differences are due to rounding off.  In real life situations the small differences would not matter.


4 lbs. 9 oz. is how many kg?

4/2.2 = 1.813 kg or 1813 mg and 9 oz. x 31 = 279 mg.

1813 mg + 279 mg = 2092 mg or 2.092 kg.

# WEIGHTS

Weight problems - there really is a reason for them. The reason is that a smaller person would probably require less medicine than a big person.

This person might get this much medicine

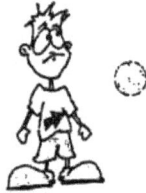

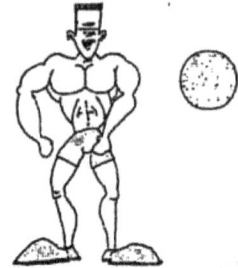

This person might get this much medicine

Because they weigh different amounts they would get different amounts of medicine. The question is how much.

If this person gets this much medicine

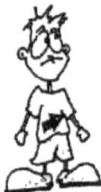

A person weighing twice as much would get twice as much

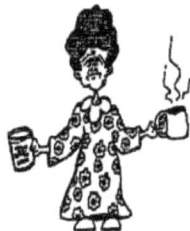

A person weighing 3 times as much would get 3 imes as much

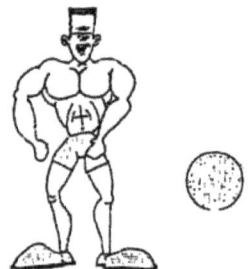

What we're really saying is that the pill the doctor ordered all disolved in the patients body gives a concentration throughout or "level".

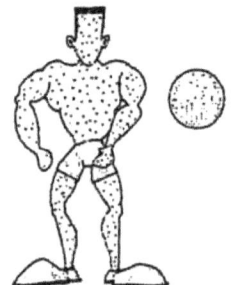

More of the same medications in the same patient's body would cause a higher level or concentration.

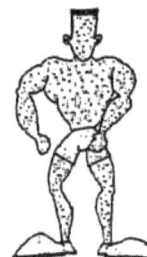

And less of the same medicine all dissolved would be a lower concentration.

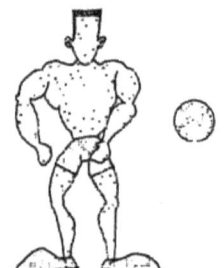

The concentration or level can be somewhat accuratley predicted by the persons weight because the human body is about 60% water.

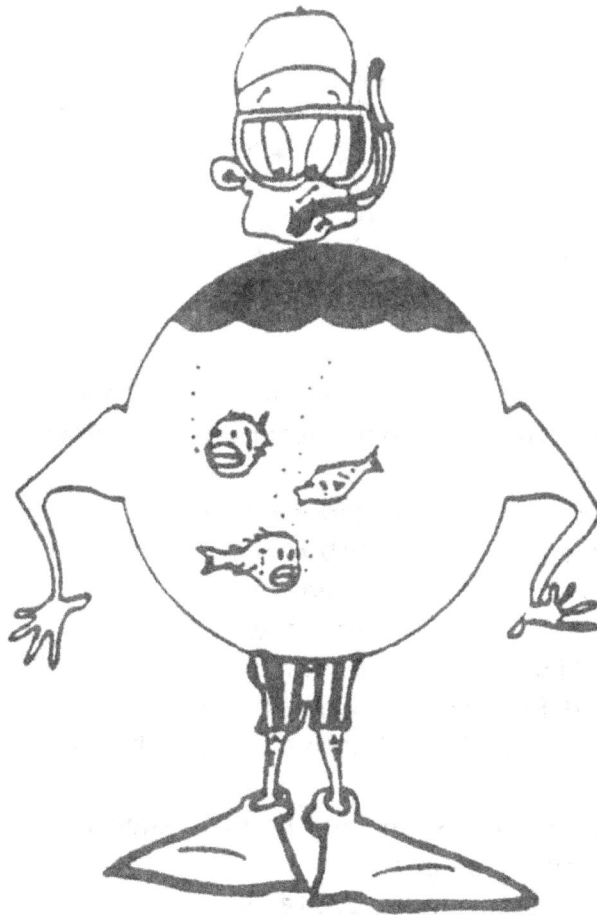

Do you remember the kool-Aid? We want the right amount of powder (medicine) for the various sizes of containers (the patient's body).

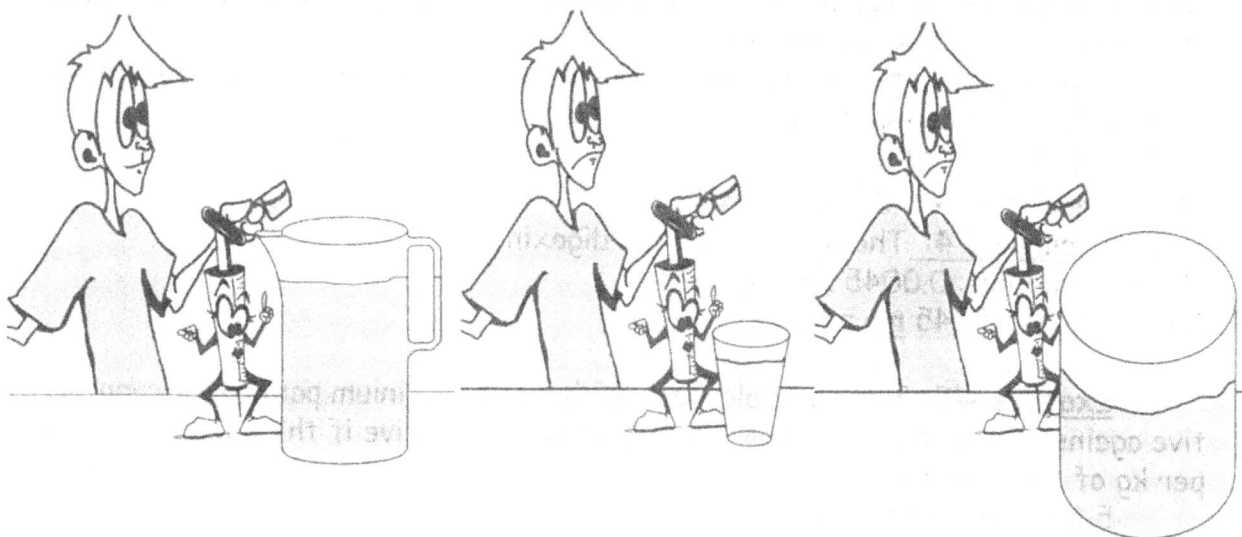

To get the level right you would match the amount of powder with the container or in other words, match the drug dosage with the patient's weight.

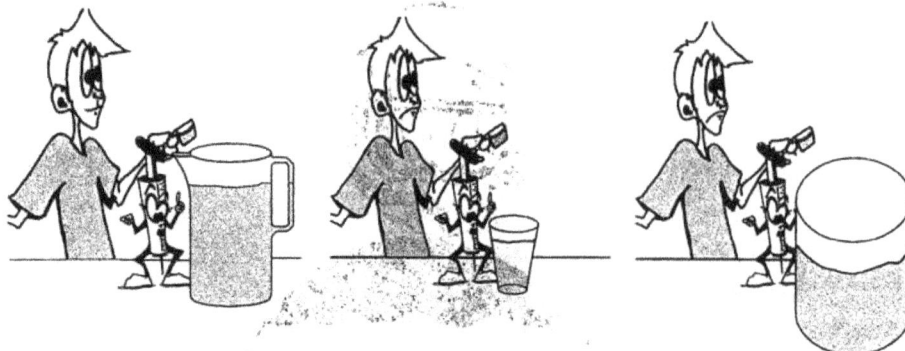

The best example I can find is not medicine but food for a premature infant. In a pediatric nursing book I found the daily nutritional requirements for a premature infant as follows:

| | |
|---|---|
| Calories | 125 kcal / kg |
| Water | 135 ml / kg |
| Protein | 4 mg / kg |
| Fat | 6gm / kg |
| Carbohydrates | 13 gm / kg |

All this means that for each kilogram the bay weighs, you would feed the baby 4 grams of protein, 6 grams of fat, 13 grams of carbohydrates and 135 milliliters of water each day.

If the baby weighed 6.6 lbs, that would be 3 kilograms (6.6 / 2.2 = 3) So you would make sure the baby got:\

$3 \times 4 = 12$ grams of proteins
$3 \times 6 = 18$ grams of fat
$3 \times 13 = 39$ grams of carbohydrate
$3 \times 135 = 405$ ml of water

<u>Example #2</u>: Bobby weighs 30 kg (66 lbs.) The doctor ordered 20 mg. of penicillin/kg per day. (That might be written: PCN 20mg / kg / day.) That means for each kilogram Bobby weighs he should receive 20 mg of penicillin. So you multiply $30 \times 20$ mg to get 600 mg per day.

<u>Example #3</u>: The doctor ordered epinephrine subcutaneously PDR (Physician's Desk Reference) instructions are: .01 mg / kg
The child's weight: 15 kg
The dose is 15 kg $\times$ 0.01 mg / kg = 0.15 mg

<u>Example #4</u>: The doctor ordered digoxin.
PDR instructions: 0.0045 mg / kg / day
Dose: 5 kg $\times$ 0.0045 $\dfrac{mg}{kg}$ = 25 mg

<u>Example #5</u>: Four year old Joe weighs 18kg. Pyrinium pamoate (Pcvan) is effective against pinworms. How many milligrams will he receive if the doctor ordered 5 mg per kg of body weight?

5 $\dfrac{mg}{kg} \times$ 18 kg = 90 mg

# PEDIATRIC DOSES

Another aspect of weights in drug calculations is pediatric doses. Where before we were calculating the dose based on the patient's weight, here we're checking the dose.

As a nurse you have a good idea of normal adult doses. You use that knowledge to give only safe doses - even though they were ordered by the doctor and issued by the pharmacy - both higher authorities. Further , when you give an unfamiliar drug its quite easy to look up the average adult dose in any drug handbook.

For instance, two 350 mg. Tylenols, 650 mg. would be o.k. for most adults. 6500 mg. or 6.5 mg. should arouse some suspicion.

In the case of children dosages vary widely bacause their sizes vary a lot. Even the same child could gain or lose a significant percentage of their weight. Consequently a pill or injection that would be therapetic in one child could be subtherapeutic in a larger child or toxic in a smaller child.

One way to check dosaages for safe quantities is to use Clark's Rule. Clark's Rule assumes an average adult weight of 150 lbs. The safe dose for a child is the same proportion to the normal adult dose as the child's weight is proportional to 150 lbs. (the normal adult weight). For instance, a 75 lb. child weighs half as much as the 150 lb. adult. So the safe dose for the child would be about half of the normal adult dose. If the child weighed 100 lbs. the safe dose would be 2/3 of the normal adult dose.

## Young's Rule

Another way to do exactly the same thing is Young's Rule. This uses the child's age to verify the quantity. It's easier to show the examples than explain it.

=================================================================================

| $\dfrac{\text{child's age}}{\text{child's age} + 12 \text{ year's}}$ | = | the number to multiply an adult dose by |
|---|---|---|
| 2 years old $\dfrac{2}{2+12} = \dfrac{2}{14} = .14$ | | multiply the adult dose by .14 to get the dose for a 2 year old |
| 3 years old $\dfrac{3}{3+12} = \dfrac{3}{15} = .2$ | | multiply the adult dose by .2 to get the dose for a 3 year old |
| 4 years old $\dfrac{4}{4+12} = \dfrac{4}{16} = .25$ | | multiply the adult dose by .25 to get the dose for a 4 year old |
| 5 year old $\dfrac{5}{5+12} = \dfrac{5}{17} = .29$ | | multiply the adult dose by .29 to get the dose for a 5 year old |
| 6 year old $\dfrac{6}{5+12} = \dfrac{6}{18} = .33$ | | multiply the adult dose by .33 to get the dose for a 6 year old |

7 years old $\dfrac{7}{7+12} = \dfrac{7}{19} = .368$      multiply the adult dose by .368 to get the dose for a 7 year old

===================================================================

8 years old $\dfrac{8}{8+12} = \dfrac{8}{20} = .4$      multiply the adult dose by .4 to get the dose for a 8 year old

===================================================================

9 years old $\dfrac{9}{9+12} = \dfrac{9}{21} = .428$      multiply the adult dose by .368 to get the dose for a 9 year old

===================================================================

10 years old $\dfrac{10}{10+12} = \dfrac{10}{22} = .454$      multiply the adult dose by .454 to get the dose for a 10 year old

===================================================================

11 years old $\dfrac{11}{11+12} = \dfrac{11}{23} = .478$      multiply the adult dose by .478 to get the dose for a 11 year old

===================================================================

12 years old $\dfrac{12}{12+12} = \dfrac{12}{24} = .5$      multiply the adult dose by .5 to get the dose for a 12 year old

===================================================================

13 years old $\dfrac{13}{13+12} = \dfrac{13}{25} = .52$      multiplty the adult dose by .52 to get the dose for a 13 year old

===================================================================

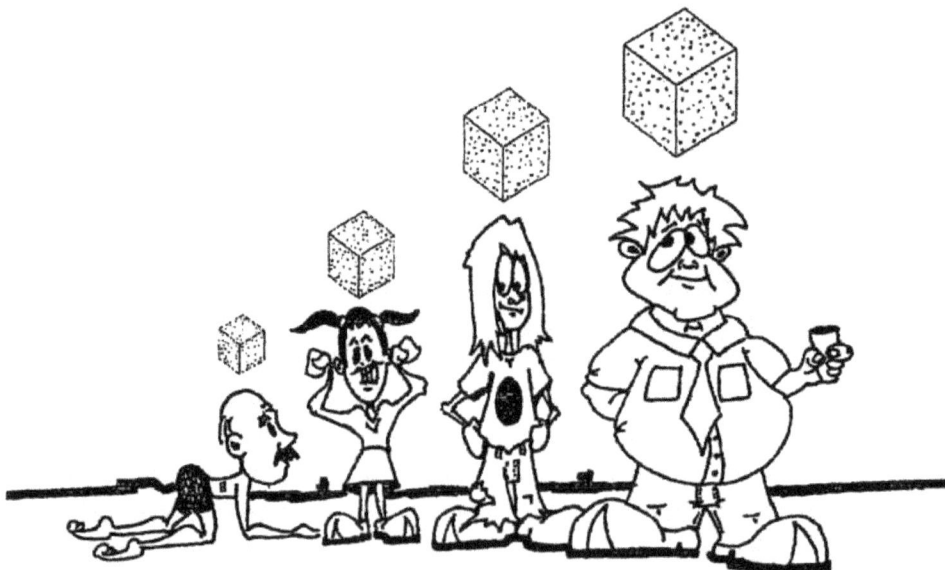

This time I really lied ...more units...grains

Grains, 61 mg. , ara a remant from the old apothecary system. I looked it up. The dictionary says it's derived from the weight of "a grain of wheat." I'm sure you also really want to know ther are 5700 grains in one pound.

By far the most common use of grains is aspirin and Tylenol. Both aspirin and Tylenol are 5 grains or 325 mg per tablet. Doctors often write, "Tylenol 10 gr P.O. q 4-6 h P.R.N. That would be two tablets. The correct abbreveation is gr.

The only other time I have seen grains is nitroglycerin sublingual - you know the little tablets to stick under someone's tongue when they are having chest pain. By far the most common stength is "1/150 gr." You can divide by yourself    1/150 gr. 61 mg/ 150 = .4mg

Doctor's frequently write "nitro 1/150 gr. p.r.n. chest pain may be repeated × 2 q 5 min if no relief."

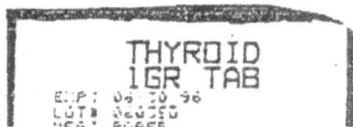

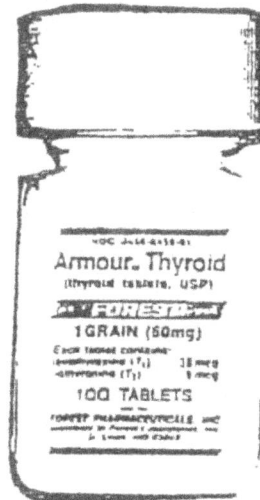

I did find one other drug measured in grains - thyroid  extract. You'll notice the bottle says 60 mg. Obviously they didn't read my book.

I lied. More units. . . micrograms

Another unit you'll frequently see is micrograms. A microgram is 1/1000 of milligram or one millionth of a gram.

That's pretty small. The correct abbreveation is **mcg**. In doctor's hand writing that could be misread as mg. Here are some examples of drugs in micrograms. by far the most frequently prescribed microgram drug is lanoxin. Tablets come in 0.250 mg and 0.500 mg or said differently 125mcg. 250mcg. 500mcg. Here are some lanoxin labels

```
LANOXIN
CALCITROL
ROCALTROL
0.25MCG CAP
EXP: 11/01/95
LOT# 102240

LANOXIN®
(DIGOXIN)

FLUDROCORTISON
ACETATE
FLORINEF
0.1MG TAB
EXP: 10/30/95
LOT# 102940

DIGOXIN
500 mcg/2 mL

MISOPROSTOL
CYTOTEC
200MCG TAB

DDAVP®
Injection
(desmopressin acetat

preservative free

10 ampules 1 mL
4 mcg/mL
```

Here is the best (most confusing) example micrograms and milligrams. Levothyroxine. The doc ordered "levonex.175 mg P.O. Q.D." The first thing I did was look up levonex because our packaging had the generic name. Then I fished through the med drawer to find one package "levothyroxine 0.075 mg."

First lets look at .175 mg. If a microgram is 1/1000 of a milligram or .001 mg, then 75 micrograms is .075 mg.

100mcg + 75mcg. = 175mcg. or .100mg + .075mg. = .175 mg

One last tip: if you ever hear a doctor talking about "a gram of dig." Jump in, interrupt, anything to say "A gram!!! Don't you mean a milligram."

```
LEVOTHYROXINE
SODIUM (0.1MG)
(LEVOTHROID)
100MCG TAB

LEVOTHYROXINE
SODIUM
LEVOTHROID
75MCG TAB

LEVOTHROID
LEVOTHYROXINE 0.15 MG TAB

LEVOTHROID
(FOR SYNTHROID
0.088MG TAB
EXP: 08/31/99
LOT# 7981
MFG: FOREST
NW MEDICAL CTR PHARMACY
```

Don't worry. This one isn't a calculation. . .**mg./hour.**

This one isn't exactly a unit. But the way doctors write it, you'd think it is a unit. Transdermal nitroglycerin is specified by the amount per hour. Here are some examples. Doctors often write "nitro-dur .4 mg." What they mean is .4mg/hour. Or they may write the total amount delivered in 24 hours. In the case of .4 mg/hour, the daily amount would be 24 hours x .4 mg/hour = 9.6 mg.

NDC-0085-3320-01      Contents: 1 unit

**INPATIENT USE ONLY**

**Nitro-Dur®**
(nitroglycerin)
Transdermal Infusion System

**0.4 mg/hr**

(20 cm²)

Each 20 cm² unit contains 80 mg of nitroglycerin.
Approximate rated release in vivo 0.4 mg/hr.
Caution: Federal law prohibits
dispensing without prescription.

Key Pharmaceuticals, Inc.
TM Kenilworth, NJ 07033 USA

NDC-0085-3310-01      Contents: 1 unit

**INPATIENT USE ONLY**

**Nitro-Dur®**
(nitroglycerin)
Transdermal Infusion System

**0.2 mg/hr**
(10 cm²)

Each 10 cm² unit contains 40 mg of nitroglycerin.
Approximate rated release in vivo 0.2 mg/hr.
Caution: Federal law prohibits dispensing
without prescription.

Key Pharmaceuticals, Inc.
TM Kenilworth, NJ 07033 USA

NDC-0085-3315-01      Contents: 1 unit

**INPATIENT USE ONLY**

**Nitro-Dur®**
(nitroglycerin)
Transdermal Infusion System

**0.3 mg/hr**

(15 cm²)

Each 15 cm² unit contains 60 mg of nitroglycerin.
Approximate rated release in vivo 0.3 mg/hr.
Caution: Federal law prohibits
dispensing without prescription.

Key Pharmaceuticals, Inc.
TM Kenilworth, NJ 07033 USA

NDC-0085-3305-01      Contents: 1 unit

**INPATIENT USE ONLY**

**Nitro-Dur®**
(nitroglycerin)
Transdermal Infusion System

**0.1 mg/hr**
(5 cm²)

Each 5 cm² unit contains 20 mg of nitroglycerin
Approximate rated release in vivo 0.1 mg/hr
Caution: Federal law prohibits dispensing
without prescription.

Pharmaceuticals, Inc.

I don't believe it. . . another unit. . .milliquivalent mEq

I asked the pharmacist to explain milliquivalents to me. She did. I didn't under-stand. It doesn't matter. The only thing you need to know is that some drugs come in **mEq.**

By far the most common is potassium. Some frequent trade names are K-lor. K-dur is a large 20 **mEq** tablet that easily splits into two halves of 10 **mEq.** each. K-lor is an orange powder (which doesn't taste too bad) that mixes in water to give 20 **mEq.** The advantage is that you can give any amount by dissolving the powder in water and taking the amount you need.

Lets say the order called for 15 mEq. of potassium. You would mix the K-lor in a comfortable amount of water. By that I mean an amount that you can measure easily and the patient can drink easily. Try 100cc which is one or two good swallows. The 100cc would have 20mEq of potassium swimming around. 20 mEq per 100cc.

$$\frac{20 \text{ mEq}}{100 \text{ cc}} = \frac{1 \text{mEq}}{5 \text{ cc}}$$    Each 5cc has 1 mEq of potassium.

So 15 mEq would be 15 x 5cc = 75cc. Another way to say it is three fourths of the potassium.

One final comment it doesn't taste bad. So don't let anyone give you a hard time about the taste.

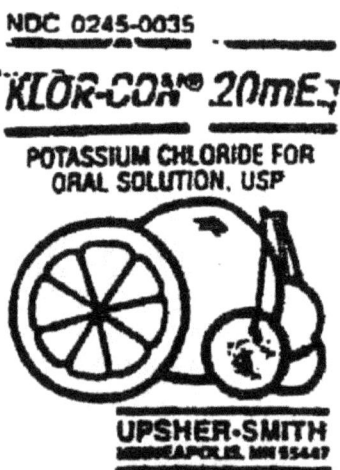

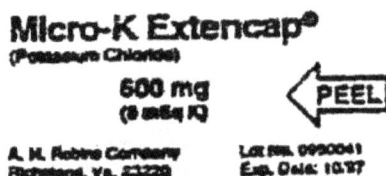

NDC 0245-0035

**KLOR-CON® 20mEq**

POTASSIUM CHLORIDE FOR
ORAL SOLUTION, USP

UPSHER-SMITH
MINNEAPOLIS, MN 55447

**Micro-K Extencap®**
(Potassium Chloride)

**600 mg**
(8 mEq K)

PEEL

A. H. Robins Company
Richmond, Va. 23220

Lot No. 0990041
Exp. Date: 10.87

# A tablespoon (tbsp) is 15cc.

# A teaspoon (tsp) is 5cc.

These quantities are still used in prescribing medications. I cannot remember which is which. I have to look it up every time. What is a tablespoon? Is it what I eat with? I don't drink tea. I don't sit at a table because I eat watching TV. If anybody has any memory devices please tell me and I add your name to all future printings.

# CRITICAL CARE CALCULATIONS

"Critical care calculations are mostly setting the I.V. rate based on the patient's weight."

The previous weight calculations we did, the pediatric doses, set the **dose** based on the patients weight. The critical care calculations we'll do set the **rate** based on the weight.

This guy would require this much medicine.

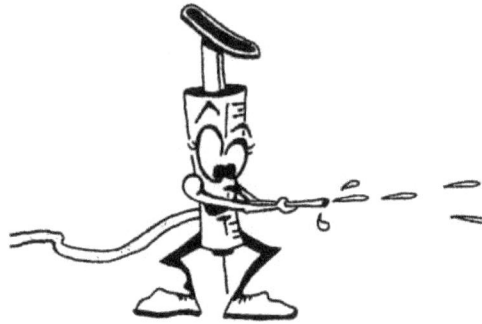

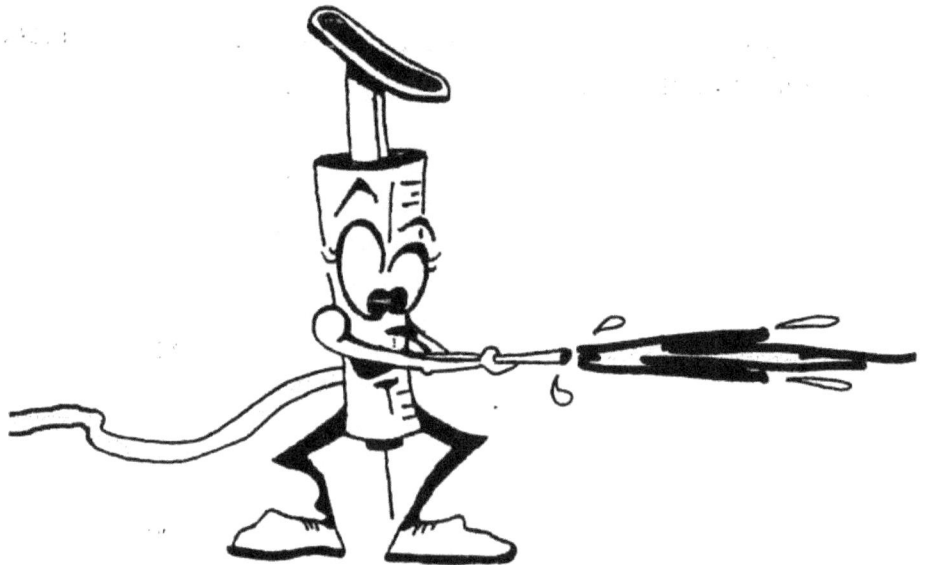

This guy would require this much medicine.

The reason is that these drugs are very quickly metabolized by the liver and kidney. So maintaining a therapeutic level is equalizing what comes in with what goes out.

Lets start with weights. Usually the first step is to convert pounds to kilograms. A kilogram weighs 2.2 lbs. And of course, the easy way to remember that is you'd rather weigh yourself in kilograms.

Reviewing quickly: A gram is 1/1000 of a gram. Two large paper clips weigh a gram. A milligram is 1/1000 of a gram. A pin weighs 50mg. A microgram is 1/1000 of a milligram. A microgram is 1/1,000,000 of a gram.

Typically critical care I.V. orders are written, "mcg./kg./min." - micrograms per kilogram per minute.

Or more clearly stated, one microgram per minute for each kilogram of body weight.

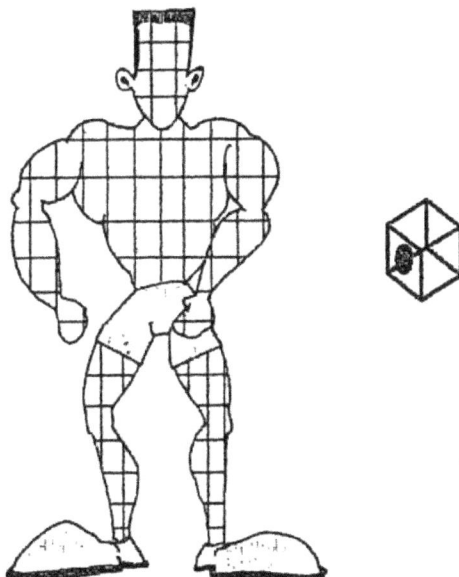

Each kilogram of body weight should have one microgram of medication flowing through it each minute.

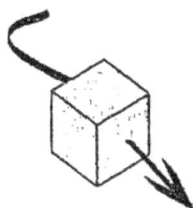

## Example #1

The doctor ordered dopamine 10 mcg/kg/min for Mr. White, a 176 lb male. The nurse mixed the infusion 800 mg of dopamine in 500 cc D5w. What is the rate to set the pump?

First: 176 lb. is 80 kg. (176/2.2 = 80). If every one of his 80 kilograms got 10 micrograms per minute we could hook up 80 I.V. lines to each kilogram. (That's a joke.) Or we could infuse 800 mcg./min. I recommend the second approach.

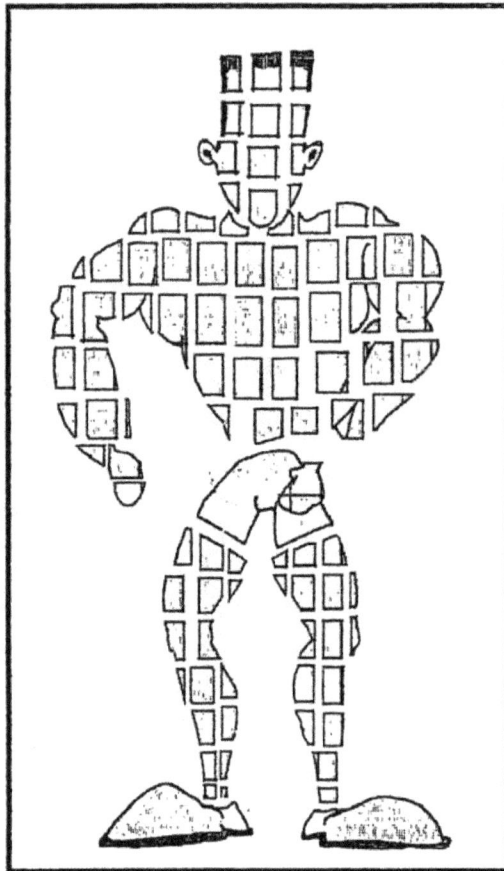

The next question is how many micrograms in each milliliter of the solution. There are 800 mg of dopamine in 500 cc of D5w. Since there are 1000 mcg. in each mg. there are 800,000 in the 500 cc. Putting that into a fraction 800,000 mcg/500 cc = 1600 mcg/cc   There are 1600 mcg in each cc of D5W. We want 800 mcg per minute. Since there are 1600 mcg in each cc. we would need 1/2 cc per minute. We would set the pump at 30 cc per hour.

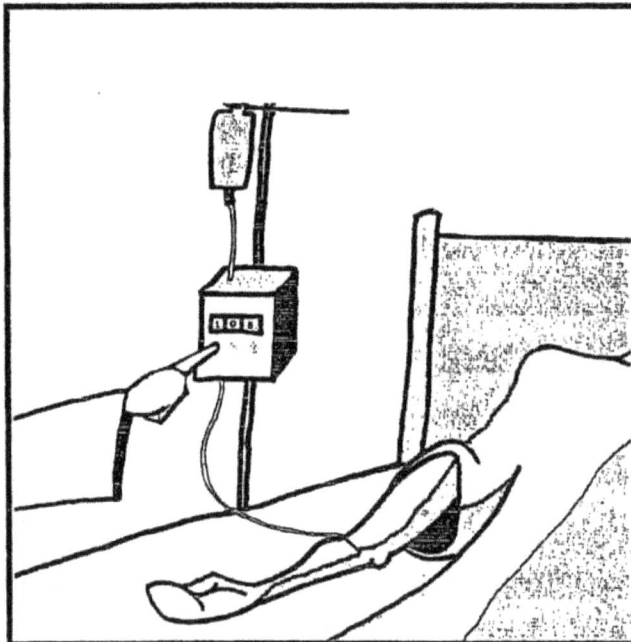

## Critical Care Example#2

Lets imagine a pretend situation that shows typical problems you'll have with critical care drips. You walk into a room. The patient is getting dobutamine (Dobutrex) 500mg in 250cc D5W make sure the rate is correct. That's not always so easy. You look through the chart and see an order from five days ago when the patient was in the unit. The original order says, "Dobutrex 5mcg/kg/min." Just by looking you estimate the patients weight at 120 to 130 pounds. At 2.2 kg per pound 55 kg would be 121 pounds - which is close. Close enough to see if you are in the ball park.

5mcg/kg/min multiplied by 55 kg is 275 micrograms per minute or 16,500 micrograms per hour (60 x 275).

The bag has 500mg of dobutamine floating around in 250cc of D5W. Each cc has 2mg floting around in it. Since there are 1000 micrograms in each milligram, there are 2000 mcg in each cc.

We want to see how many those cc's to infuse per hour to give 16,500 mcg per hour. I calculate 8.25 cc/hr. Since the pump can't be adjusted to fractions, we would round off to 8cc/hr. THE PUMP WAS RUNNING AT 3CC/HR!!!! That is not even close to 8cc/hr.

Way off. Where do we start? First lets get an exact weight. You do that. 118 pounds. You're close there. Next consider that dobutamine's intended or unintended effect would show up in the blood pressure. So you look back over the vitial sign flow sheets to see if the blood pressure had significantly changed in five days. However you see that it has been fairly constant.

Next you go over intake/output to see I.V. flow rates over the past five days. You notice four days ago, in the intensive care unit, the rate was changed from 5cc/hr to 3cc/hr. Hmmmmm. Looking closer at the ICU notes shows the concentration, originally at 5cc/hr, was 1000mg of dobutamine in 250cc D5W. You see at this point the concentration was changed to 500mg in 250cc when the rate was changed to 3cc/hr. Very suspicious.

Lets look at 1 gram (1000mg) dobutamine in 250cc D5W at 5cc/hr. 1000mg in 250cc is 4mg per cc or 4000mcg per cc, 5 of these cc's an hour is 20mg/hr (20,000mcg/hr) or 333mcg/min (I got that by dividing 20,000by 60). If we divide 333mcg/min by 55kg (his weight) we get 6mcg/kg/min. So the initial rate was probably set based on a few more pounds. Then when they cut the concentration in half, they cut the rate in half instead of DOUBLING it.

Example #3

For some reason the doctor specified Procainamide 500mg in 100cc D5W at 2mg/min. 2mg/min is very standard for Pronestyl. That concentration is quite unusual. Why doctors specify the mix concentration I don't know. The delivery (2mg/min) is the only thing that matters.

Most commonly procainamide is mixed 2 grams in 250cc. As we saw in the last problem that concentration is 8mg per cc. Any other concentration confuses the issue and likely sets up mistakes.

You come on and see Pronestyl 500mg in 250cc D%W at 10cc/hr. you see on the clip board - the following sheet which clearly states "2grams in 250 cc", that's a bad sign.

So just the same way as we figured out the standard drip, we'll figure out the hourly rate on the pump for the specified 2mg/min. If there are 500mg in 100cc there are 5mg in each cc.
If we want 2mg/min - that's the same as 120mg/hour. To get 120mg we need 24cc. To get 120mg/hour we need to set the pump at 24cc/hour.

Normally the pharmacy would call the doctor and explain the high potential for mistakes. And they usually agree to the standard mixtures. If they don't then the pharmacy will attach a sticker that warns of an unusual mixture.

## MAINTAIN

## ACCURATE

## RATE

LIDOCAINE/PRONESTYL/BRETYLOL:

| 2GM / 100cc | 2GM / 250cc |
|---|---|
| 60cc - 4mg/min | 60cc - 4mg/min |
| 45cc - 3mg/min | 45cc - 4mg/min |
| 30cc - 2mg/min | 22cc - 1/min |
| 15cc - 1mg/min | 15cc - 1mg/min |

# Critical Care Example #4

Nitroglycerine is given I.V. in ongoing heart attacks. Like all nitrates it opens arteries. That's a great thing to do for an M.I. I've mostly seen 50mg of nitro mixed in 250cc D5W (always in a glass bottle). The intended effect is to dilate coronary arteries.

The unintended effect is to dilate all arteries and significantly lower blood pressure. Doctors generally want to give as mush nitro as they can without dropping the blood pressure too much. A typical order might be: "Titrate Nitro to keep systolic blood pressure above 100. Start at 10 mics." That means increase the nitro drip rate until the blood pressure falls to 100 mm Hg systolic. Lets find out what "10 mics" means.

Lets keep going. You see the nurse following up on the order, starting the drip rate at 3cc/hr on the pump. You ask very casually, "How many mic's is the patient getting?" She says, "Ten."

Lets look closer. 50mg of nitro in 250cc D5W. That's 50,000 micrograms in 250cc of D5W. In each cc there are 200mcg. I got that by dividing 50,000mcg by 250cc. Setting the pump at one cc per hour would infuse 200mcg/hr. Since there are 60 minutes in an hour that would be 3.3mcg/min. 3.3 micrograms are infusing each minute. Setting the pump at 3cc/hr would infusing 9.9mcg/min. So they aren't wrong to say ten. Increasing the pump rate by each cc/hr would increase the nitro infusion by 3.3

# Nitroglycerin infusion

## 50 mg Ntg/250 cc 5D/W =200 mcg/cc

3 cc/hr = 10 mcg/min

6cc/hr = 20 mcg/min

9cc/hr = 30 mcg/min

12cc/hr = 40 mcg/min

15cc/hr = 50 mcg/min

18cc/hr = 60 mcg/min

21cc/hr = 70 mcg/min

24cc/hr = 80 mcg/min

27cc/hr = 90 mcg/min

30cc/hr = 100mcg/min

etc.

(maxium dose is 200 mcg/min)

\* Always make sure B/P is stable before titrating higher.

# Example #5

Let's look at this Nitro bottle. You'll notice the label is also written upside down (because the bottle is hung upside down). 100mg in 250ml is .4mg (400mcg) per ml. They tell you that on the label. You could do the division 100mg/250ml = .4mg/ml. How many mics/min would the patient be getting if the I.V. pump is 23ml/hour?

$$\frac{23ml}{hour} \times \frac{400mcg}{ml} \times \frac{1\ hour}{60\ min} = 153\ \frac{mics}{min}$$

At my hospital where they use **this** concentration there is a calculation factor of 6.6 which coincidentally is 400/60. So you could get the same answer by multiplying 23 x 6.6. But watch the concentration carefully.

1A0696
NDC 0338-1051-02

**Baxter**

250 mL

100 mg
Nitroglycerin
in 5% Dextrose
Injection
(400 mcg/mL)

Each 100 mL contains 40 mg of Nitroglycerin (added as Diluted Nitroglycerin, USP with propylene glycol), 5 g Dextrose Hydrous, USP, 0.84 mL Alcohol, USP (added as a dissolution aid) and 108 mg Citric Acid Hydrous, USP added as a buffer. pH adjusted with sodium hydroxide and if necessary hydrochloric acid. pH 4.0 (3.0 to 5.0). Hypertonic. 465 mOsmol/L (calc). Sterile. Single dose container. Dosage: For intravenous use. Use only if vacuum is present and solution is clear. Administration set can

exact amount of nitroglycerin delivered to patient. See insert. Caution: Do not add supplementary medication. Do not administer simultaneously with blood. Federal (USA) law prohibits dispensing without prescription. Storage: Room temperature (25°C). Avoid excessive heat. Protect from freezing. See insert. For Product Information 1-800-933-0303 Baxter Healthcare Corporation Deerfield, IL 60015 USA Made in USA

100 mg Nitroglycerin in
5% Dextrose Injection (400 mcg/mL)

Example #6

Where I used to work they have a file of these ridiculous charts.
When I tried to use it I couldn't figure it out.  Actually, a
nurse who had traded me a Memorial weekend Saturday for the
previous Thursday asked me to check her calculation and gave me
this chart.  I ended up figuring it out the same old way and then
working backwards on the stupid chart.

So here it goes: 5kg/kg/min for a 75 pound patient.  (1) 5
micrograms per kilogram times 75 kilograms is 375 micrograms per
minute.  (2) 375 micrograms per minute is 22,500 micrograms per
hour.

(1)   $\dfrac{5 \text{ mcg}}{\text{kg/min}} \times 75\text{kg} = \dfrac{375 \text{ mcg}}{\text{min}}$

(2)   $\dfrac{375 \text{ mcg}}{\text{min}} \times \dfrac{60 \text{ min}}{\text{hour}} = 22{,}000 \dfrac{\text{mcg}}{\text{hr}}$

(3)   If there are 1.6mg of dopamine in each ml "400mg in 250ml",
      there are 1600mcg in each ml.

      $22{,}500 \dfrac{\text{mcg}}{\text{hour}} \times \dfrac{\text{ml}}{1600\text{mcg}} = 14\text{cc/hour}$

Now just figure that out on the stupid chart.

(1)   Look up the weight.
(2)   Go down the column under 75kg to 5.3 (close to 5).
(3)   Follow that line left to the end where it says "15"
      which is close to 14.

### Dopamine Solution (Intropin) 1,600 mcg/ml
#### (800 mg Intropin/500 ml or 400 mg Intropin/250 ml)

| Flow Rate mcgtt/minute | Quantity of Dopamine mcg/*minute | Body Weight | | | | | | | | | | | | | | | |
|---|---|---|---|---|---|---|---|---|---|---|---|---|---|---|---|---|---|
| | | lb | 77 | 88 | 99 | 110 | 121 | 132 | 143 | 154 | 165 | 176 | 187 | 198 | 209 | 220 | 231 | 242 |
| | | kg | 35 | 40 | 45 | 50 | 55 | 60 | 65 | 70 | 75 | 80 | 85 | 90 | 95 | 100 | 105 | 110 |
| 5 | 133 | | 3.8 | 3.4 | 2.9 | 2.6 | 2.4 | 2.2 | 2.0 | 1.9 | 1.8 | 1.6 | 1.6 | 1.5 | 1.4 | 1.3 | 1.3 | 1.2 |
| 10 | 267 | | 7.6 | 6.7 | 5.9 | 5.3 | 4.9 | 4.5 | 4.1 | 3.8 | 3.6 | 3.3 | 3.1 | 3.0 | 2.8 | 2.7 | 2.5 | 2.4 |
| 15 | 400 | | 11 | 10 | 8.9 | 8.0 | 7.3 | 6.6 | 6.1 | 5.7 | 5.3 | 5.0 | 4.7 | 4.4 | 4.2 | 4.0 | 3.8 | 3.6 |
| 20 | 533 | | 15 | 13 | 12 | 11 | 9.7 | 8.9 | 8.2 | 7.6 | 7.1 | 6.7 | 6.3 | 5.9 | 5.6 | 5.3 | 5.1 | 4.9 |
| 25 | 667 | | 19 | 17 | 15 | 13 | 12 | 11 | 10 | 9.5 | 8.9 | 8.4 | 7.8 | 7.4 | 7.0 | 6.6 | 6.3 | 6.0 |
| 30 | 800 | | 23 | 20 | 18 | 16 | 15 | 13 | 12 | 11 | 11 | 10 | 9.4 | 8.9 | 8.4 | 8.0 | 7.6 | 7.3 |
| 35 | 933 | | 27 | 23 | 21 | 19 | 17 | 16 | 14 | 13 | 12 | 12 | 11 | 10 | 9.8 | 9.3 | 8.9 | 8.5 |
| 40 | 1067 | | 31 | 27 | 24 | 21 | 19 | 18 | 16 | 15 | 14 | 13 | 13 | 12 | 11 | 11 | 10 | 9.7 |
| 45 | 1200 | | 34 | 30 | 27 | 24 | 22 | 20 | 18 | 17 | 16 | 15 | 14 | 13 | 13 | 12 | 11 | 11 |
| 50 | 1333 | | 38 | 33 | 30 | 27 | 24 | 22 | 21 | 19 | 18 | 17 | 16 | 15 | 14 | 13 | 13 | 12 |
| 55 | 1467 | | 42 | 37 | 33 | 29 | 27 | 24 | 23 | 21 | 20 | 18 | 17 | 16 | 15 | 15 | 14 | 13 |
| 60 | 1600 | | 46 | 40 | 36 | 32 | 29 | 27 | 25 | 23 | 21 | 20 | 19 | 18 | 17 | 16 | 15 | 15 |
| 65 | 1733 | | 50 | 43 | 39 | 35 | 32 | 29 | 27 | 25 | 23 | 22 | 20 | 19 | 18 | 17 | 17 | 16 |
| 70 | 1867 | | 53 | 47 | 42 | 37 | 34 | 31 | 29 | 27 | 25 | 23 | 22 | 21 | 20 | 19 | 18 | 17 |
| 75 | 2000 | | 57 | 50 | 45 | 40 | 36 | 33 | 31 | 29 | 27 | 25 | 24 | 22 | 21 | 20 | 19 | 18 |
| 80 | 2133 | | 61 | 53 | 47 | 43 | 39 | 36 | 33 | 31 | 28 | 27 | 25 | 24 | 23 | 21 | 20 | 19 |
| 85 | 2267 | | 65 | 57 | 50 | 45 | 41 | 38 | 35 | 32 | 30 | 28 | 27 | 25 | 24 | 23 | 22 | 21 |
| 90 | 2400 | | 69 | 60 | 53 | 48 | 44 | 40 | 37 | 34 | 32 | 30 | 28 | 27 | 25 | 24 | 23 | 22 |
| 95 | 2533 | | 72 | 63 | 56 | 51 | 46 | 42 | 39 | 36 | 34 | 32 | 29 | 28 | 27 | 25 | 24 | 23 |
| 100 | 2667 | | 76 | 67 | 59 | 53 | 49 | 45 | 41 | 38 | 36 | 33 | 31 | 30 | 28 | 27 | 25 | 24 |

dosage = mcg dopamine/kg/minute

*based on 60 mcgtt/ml, each mcgtt of this solution contains 26.7 mcg dopamine

titration guidelines:                       Selected side effects/contraindications:

Example #7

**This is another method.** If you have similar charts on your clipboards, they can be very helpful. If the concentration is the same and the rate is listed you can simply divide the mics/kg given by the patients weight.

For instance, Dopamine 800mg in 250cc @ 20cc is 1066mcg/min. If your patient weighs 70kg, that works out to 15mics/kg/min.

If the rate is not on the list than lets say dopamine 250mg/800cc @ 13cc/hour. Start @ 1cc: that's 54mcg/min. Multiply that by 13 for 702 mcg. Then divide by the weight, 70kg, which is 10 mcg/min/kg.

**CONVERSION CHART**

**DOPAMINE:**

| 800mg / 250cc | 400mg / 250cc<br>800mg / 500cc |
|---|---|
| 60cc = 3200mcg/min | 60cc = 1600mcg/min |
| 50cc = 2666mcg/min | 50cc = 1333mcg/min |
| 40cc = 2134mcg/min | 40cc = 1067mcg/min |
| 30cc = 1600mcg/min | 30cc = 800mcg/min |
| 20cc = 1066mcg/min | 20cc = 533mcg/min |
| 15cc = 800mcg/min | 15cc = 400mcg/min |
| 10cc = 534mcg/min | 10cc = 267mcg/min |
| 5cc = 266mcg/min | 5cc = 133mcg/min |
| 3cc = 160mcg/min | 3cc = 80mcg/min |
| 2cc = 106mcg/min | 2cc = 53mcg/min |
| 1cc = 54mcg/min | 1cc = 27mcg/min |

# CALC FACTOR
## Another Way

There is another way to do exactly the same thing, except it's easier to remember. When you walk into a room, look at the pump and need to quickly calculate the mic's per kg per minute try this method:

#1:   The "calc factor" - the drug in the solution
       Dopamine 800mg in 250cc D5W          800/250 = 3.2
       Dopamine 800mg in 500cc D5W          800/500 = 1.6
       Isuprel 8mg in 500 D5W                 8/500 =  .0016
       Dobutamine 2 grams in 250 D5W      2000/250 = 8

#2:   Multiply by 1000

#3:   Multiply by the rate the pump is going

#4:   Divide by the weight in kilograms

#5:   Divide by 60

## Example #8
### Dobutrex 5 mics

The patient weighs 74 kg. Dobutrex we mix 500mg in 250cc D5W. First of all, Dobutrex is 250mg in 20cc, 500mg is 40cc. I am pointing out here that squirting 40cc into 250cc would substantially change the concentration. You would have 500mg in 290cc. So you have to withdraw 40cc from the bag before you add the Dobutrex. In general it's always a good idea to withdraw the amount you are going to add. So assuming we have 500mg in 250cc we get the calc factor of $\frac{500}{250}$ x $\frac{1000}{60 \times 74}$ = .45

The calc factor times the rate is the "mics." So .45 x rate = 5. So the rate to set the pump is 11cc/hr.

Example #9
"Nitropress 50mg in 250cc D5W @ 1 mic"

We look up a starting rate for Nitropress. It says 1mcg/kg/min.
We want 1mcg/kg/min and the patient weighs 130kg. That means
for each kg we want 1mcg each minute for each kilogram. That's
130mcg each minute or 60 x 130 mcg each hour or 7800 mcg each
hour. Since there are 2mg or 200mcg per ml we would set the
pump at 39cc/hour (7800mcg/hour – 200mcg/ml).

Setting it up algebraically:

$$\frac{.2mg}{ml} \quad \frac{1000mcg}{mg} \quad \frac{1\ hour}{60\ min} \quad \frac{1}{130\ kg} \quad x \quad \frac{?ml}{hour} \quad = \quad \frac{1mcg}{kg\ min}$$

If you remember calc factor. That's exactly the same thing.

$$\frac{50}{250} \quad x \quad \frac{1000}{60\ x\ 130} \quad = CF = 0.0256$$

CF x rate = mcg/kg min

So 0.0256 x rate = 1  (rate = 39)

NITROPRESS®
Sodium Nitroprusside Inj.

50 mg/2 mL Vial
(25 mg/mL)

For I.V. infusion only.
Must be diluted.

$156.46 \, Kg$

$156$

$$156.46 \, \frac{5 \, mics}{Kg \, m} = \frac{780 \, mic}{min}$$

$$\frac{5}{780} \quad \frac{4}{780}$$
$$\frac{}{60}$$

$$\frac{46,800.}{hour}$$

$$250\overline{)400} \quad \frac{400 \, mg}{250 e}$$
$$\underline{250}$$
$$\overline{1500}$$
$$1500$$

$$\frac{46,800 \, mg}{hour}$$

$$\frac{46.8 \, mg}{hour} \quad \frac{cc}{1.6 mg}$$

$$\frac{29 \, cc}{hour}$$

$$1.6\overline{)46.8} \,/hour$$
$$\underline{32}$$
$$\overline{148}$$

On the last page you see my actual scribbles on a computer simulation of a paper towel. The reason the page looks like this is to illustrate a little more vividly what happened and not just show another example problem.

I did the calculations on a paper towel. But it didn't look like a paper towel when I photocopied the original work to print in this book. So I asked my friend Mat Kohn of Kohn Creative, a full service add agency, kohncreative.com, to make it look like the original.

The charge nurse who knew I had written this book asked me to calculate the pump rate for a patient at "5 mics".

This was on a telemetry floor and I had not worked in ICU for six months which is to say I had no cheat sheets or a sense of normal number for a dopamine drip or calc factors let alone the patient's weight of over 300 pounds and felt my own self-imposed pressure to come through. What I did is what this book tries to promote, looking at the information you have and thinking about how that information can get you to what's needed.

In the upper left corner is the weight. 156.46 kg, heavy.

$$\text{Then } 156 \text{ kg} \times \frac{5 \text{ mics}}{\text{Kg-min}} = \frac{780 \text{ mics}}{\text{min}}$$

which is $\frac{46{,}800 \text{ mics}}{\text{hour}}$

The bag of dopamine has 400mg in 250cc which is $1.6 \frac{\text{mg}}{\text{cc}}$

$\frac{46{,}800 \text{ mics}}{\text{hour}}$ is $\frac{46.8 \text{ mg}}{\text{hour}}$     (Divide by 1000.)

If each cc contains 1.6mg then 46.8 mg would be contained 29.3 cc. Set the pump at 29.3 cc/hr.

# Primacor(.5mcg/kg/min)
## Patient weighs 84kg


Primacor is a cardiac stimulant. It is usually prescribed in mcg/kg/min. Here we'll see three ways to set the drip rate. Usually it is mixed 50mg in 250cc of D5W. You'll notice on the chart they say to add "50mg (two 20ml vials and one 10ml vial)in 200ml dextrose or saline."

The easiest way is to look at a chart. Looking under the 85kg column and across on the .50mcg/kg/min you see the flow rate is 12.75ml/hour. Some pumps can be set to hundredths. Others have to be rounded off.

The next way we'll do is via algebra.

$$\frac{.5mcg}{kg\text{-}min} \times 84kg \times \frac{60\ min}{hour} \times \frac{250ml}{50mg} \times \frac{mg}{1000mcg} = \frac{12.6ml}{hour}$$

To make that long equation easier to grasp, we can break it down into smaller chunks: $\dfrac{.5mcg}{Kg\text{-}min} \times 84kg = \dfrac{42mcg}{min}$

Since there are 60 minutes in each hour we would multiply by 60 to get the micrograms per hour: 2520 mcg/hour. Since there are 50mg in 250ml, there are 50,000mcg in 250ml or 200mcg in each ml. We multiply (2520mcg/hr. x ml/200mcg) the micrograms per hour times the milliliters per microgram to get ml/hr or 12.6ml/hr. That is the rate you would set the pump.

Here's a way to check your calculations. This is very important because calculations in the ICU are often made under very stressful life and death circumstances. So to have confidence in your numbers it is good to have a double check method.

## Step #1
Multiply the mic's per minute by the weight and multiply that times 60 (60 minutes in an hour) and round off to do it quickly.

$$\frac{.5\ mics}{kg\text{-}min} \times 80kg \times \frac{60\ min}{hour} = 2400\ mcg/hour$$

## Step #2
The concentration is 50mg in 250cc, 50mg/250ml

$$\frac{50,000mcg}{250ml} = 200mcg/ml$$

Step #3
Divide the mic's per hour by the micrograms per ml.

$$\frac{2400mcg/hour}{200mcg/ml} = 12ml/hour$$

Look at it like this:

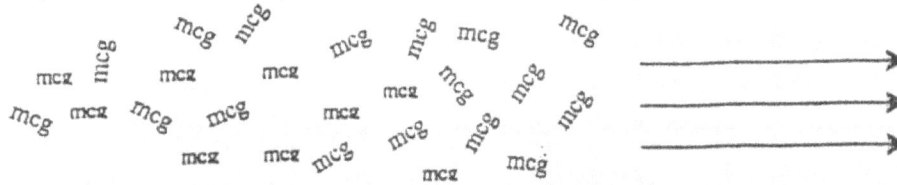

2400mcg each hour and there are 200mcg in each ml so we would need 12ml each hour.

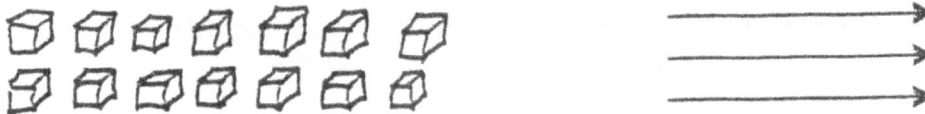

PRIMACOR milrinone lactate injection    DOSING CHARTS

DOSAGE FORMS: Undiluted — 10 mL and 20 mL single-dose vials and 5 mL sterile cartridge units
Diluted — 100 mL and 200 mL prefilled bags with 5% dextrose injection, USP

LOADING DOSE: 50 mcg/kg administered slowly over 10 minutes

Note: When using the prefilled bag for the loading dose, flow rate must be adjusted after 10 minutes (an electronic pump is recommended).

| Patient Weight (kg) | 40 | 45 | 50 | 55 | 60 | 65 | 70 | 75 | 80 | 85 | 90 | 95 | 100 | 105 | 110 |
|---|---|---|---|---|---|---|---|---|---|---|---|---|---|---|---|
| (lb) | 88 | 99 | 110 | 121 | 132 | 143 | 154 | 165 | 176 | 187 | 198 | 209 | 220 | 231 | 242 |
| Undiluted—Vials and Cartridge Units (1 mg/mL)  Loading Dose (mL) | 2.00 | 2.25 | 2.50 | 2.75 | 3.00 | 3.25 | 3.50 | 3.75 | 4.00 | 4.25 | 4.50 | 4.75 | 5.00 | 5.25 | 5.50 |
| Diluted—Prefilled Bag (0.2 mg/mL)  Loading Dose (mL) | 10.00 | 11.25 | 12.50 | 13.75 | 15.00 | 16.25 | 17.50 | 18.75 | 20.00 | 21.25 | 22.50 | 23.75 | 25.00 | 26.25 | 27.50 |

MAINTENANCE DOSE: For PRIMACOR concentration of 200 mcg/mL

PRIMACOR: 100 mL or 200 mL bag premixed with 5% dextrose injection, USP   or   50 mg (two 20 mL vials and one 10 mL vial) in 200 mL dextrose or saline (yields 50 mg/250 mL)

| Patient Weight (kg) | 40 | 45 | 50 | 55 | 60 | 65 | 70 | 75 | 80 | 85 | 90 | 95 | 100 | 105 | 110 |
|---|---|---|---|---|---|---|---|---|---|---|---|---|---|---|---|
| (lb) | 88 | 99 | 110 | 121 | 132 | 143 | 154 | 165 | 176 | 187 | 198 | 209 | 220 | 231 | 242 |
| Minimum Dose 0.375 mcg/kg/min  Flow Rate (mL/h) | 4.50 | 5.06 | 5.63 | 6.19 | 6.75 | 7.31 | 7.88 | 8.44 | 9.00 | 9.56 | 10.13 | 10.69 | 11.25 | 11.81 | 12.38 |
| Standard Dose 0.50 mcg/kg/min  Flow Rate (mL/h) | 6.00 | 6.75 | 7.50 | 8.25 | 9.00 | 9.75 | 10.50 | 11.25 | 12.00 | 12.75 | 13.50 | 14.25 | 15.00 | 15.75 | 16.50 |
| Maximum Dose 0.75 mcg/kg/min  Flow Rate (mL/h) | 9.00 | 10.13 | 11.25 | 12.38 | 13.50 | 14.63 | 15.75 | 16.88 | 18.00 | 19.13 | 20.25 | 21.38 | 22.50 | 23.63 | 24.75 |

# RULE OF SIXES

*"How much medicine in 100 ml. to provide 1 mcg/kg/min @ 1 ml/hr"*

By the rule of sixes we mix a solution so each ml/hour on the pump provides 1 mcg/kg/min. That way you know exactly how much medicine is infusing and you can adjust the amount quickly and accurately. Well start with 100 ml. volume.

6 x patient's weight (kg.) = mg. in 100 ml. solution

Example: The patient (a child) weighs 12.5 kg
6 x 12.5 = 75 mg
In a 100 ml. bag there will be 75 mg.

$$\frac{75 \text{ mg.}}{100 \text{ ml}} = \frac{75{,}000 \text{ mcg.}}{100 \text{ ml.}} = \frac{750 \text{mcg.}}{\text{ml.}}$$

$$750 \frac{\text{mcg.}}{\text{ml.}} \times \frac{\textbf{1 ml.}}{\textbf{hour}} \times \frac{1}{12.5 \text{ kg.}} \times \frac{1 \text{ hour}}{60 \text{ min}} \times = \frac{\textbf{1 mcg}}{\textbf{kg/min.}}$$

That was just to give you a general idea of the concept. Now we'll do the same problem with dopamine which comes in a vial 40 mg/ml.

6 x patient's weight (kg.) = # mg. in 100 ml. solution

Example: The patient (a child) weighs 12.5 kg. 6 x 12.5 = 75 mg.
In a 100 ml. syringe there will be 75 mg.
Dopamine comes in a vial 40mg/ml

$$\frac{75\text{mg}}{? \text{ ml.}} = \frac{40\text{mg}}{\text{ml.}} \qquad 75\text{mg.} = 1.89 \text{ ml.}$$

Withdraw 1.89 ml. from the 100 ml, bag.
Squirt in 1.89 ml. so the volume is 100 ml.

$$\frac{75 \text{ mg}}{100 \text{ ml.}} = \frac{75{,}000 \text{ mcg}}{100 \text{ ml.}} = \frac{750 \text{ mcg}}{\text{ml.}}$$

$$750 \frac{\text{mcg}}{\text{ml.}} \times \frac{1 \text{ ml.}}{\text{hour}} \times \frac{1}{12.5 \text{ kg}} \times \frac{1 \text{ hour}}{60 \text{ min}} = \frac{1\text{mcg}}{\text{kg/min}}$$

# Rule of Sixes  Dopamine so 1 ml/hour = 10 mcg/kg/min

The neonate weighs 0.7 kg
 Again we are working with the rule of sixes for a 100 ml. mixture.
To get the number of mg. of medicine to add to 100 ml. multiply the patient's weight by 6.    0.7 kg. x 6 = 4.2 mg.
Since we want **1 ml/hr** = **10 mcg/kg/min** (not 1 mcg/kg/min) multiply 4.2 x 10 =42 mg.

Dopamine comes in a vial 40 mg./ml.

$$\frac{42mg.}{? ml} = \frac{40mg.}{1 ml.} \qquad 42mg. = 1.05 ml.$$

Withdraw 1.05 ml. from the 100cc and add 1.05 ml. (42 mg.) of dopamine to the bag.

The mixture will infuse 10 mcg/kg/ml for each ml/hr on the pump.

# Rule of Sixes with a 50 ml. Syringe or Bag

We can also use a 50 ml. bag or syringe. In the last problem we used a 100 ml, bag, multiplied the patient's weight by six, added that many mg. to the bag and blah blah blah blah.....and we intended to infuse 1 ml/hr for 10 mcg/kg./min. Since 1ml/hr would last over four days, it would be more sensible and economical to use a 50 ml. bag or syringe.

Since the 50 ml. bag is one half the 100 ml bag we would add one half the medication.

For 100 ml.:   0.7 kg. x  6  = 4.2 mg.
For  50  ml.:    ½  of that amount 2.1 mg.

In the last few problems we have seen the rule of sixes with 1 mcg/kg./min, 10 mcg/kg/min, 100 ml. and 50 ml. The principle is the same.

This table should illustrate the variation with the rule of sixes

|  |  | 50 ml. | 100ml. | Rate |
|---|---|---|---|---|
| Dose | 0.01mcg/kg/min | Wt. x 0.03 | Wt. x 0.06 | 1 ml./hr. |
| Dose | 0.1 mcg/kg/min | Wt. x 0.3 | Wt. x 0.6 | 1 ml/hr |
| Dose | 1 mcg/kg/min | Wt. x 3 | Wt. x 6 | 1 ml/hr |

For CHF: " **Natrecor, Bolus 2 mcg/kg then drip 0.01mcg/kg/min.**"
The patient weighs 106 kg.

The point of this example problem is how to accurately dose extremely small amounts of medication. 0.01 mcg. is one hundred millionth of a gram (1/100,000,000) To do this the manufacturer specifies the dilution, 1.5 mg. in 250 ml.

Natrecor comes 1.5 mg. of powder in a vial. It has to be reconstituted. Withdraw 10 ml. from the 250 ml. IV bag which you will use and squirt it into the vial. Withdraw the reconstituted 10 ml. from the vial and squirt it back into the bag. That way the bag still has 250 ml. If you reconstituted the powder with sterile water and added it to the bag, there would be 260 ml. which is a volume 4% more than 250 ml. and a concentration 4% less.

What is the concentration?

$$\frac{1.5 \text{ mg.}}{250 \text{ ml.}} = \frac{1500 \text{ mcg.}}{250 \text{ ml.}} = \frac{0.006 \text{ mg.}}{\text{ml.}} = \frac{6 \text{ mcg.}}{\text{ml}}$$

The bolus: 2mcg/kg. Since you know the exact concentration of the bag, draw the bolus from the bag.

2 mcg./kg. x 106 kg. = 212 mcg. There are 6 mcg. In each ml.

For 212 mcg: $\frac{212 \text{ mcg.}}{6 \text{ mcg/ml.}}$ = 35.3 ml.

The drip: 0.01 mcg/kg./min. The patient weighs 106 kg.

106 kg. x $\frac{0.01 \text{ mg}}{\text{kg./min.}}$ = $\frac{1.06 \text{ mcg.}}{\text{Min}}$

Since there are 60 minutes in an hour, multiply by 60 to get the rate in hours.

$\frac{60 \text{ min.}}{\text{hour}}$ x $\frac{1.06 \text{ mcg.}}{\text{min.}}$ = $\frac{63.6 \text{ mcg.}}{\text{hour}}$

There are 6 mcg. In each ml.

For $\dfrac{63.3 \text{ mcg.}}{\text{hour}}$ : $\dfrac{63.3 \text{ mcg./hour}}{6 \text{ mcg./ml.}} = \dfrac{10.6 \text{ ml.}}{\text{hour}}$

$\dfrac{0.01 \text{ mcg.} \times 106 \text{ kg.} \times 60 \text{ min/hour}}{Kg - min \quad 6 \text{ mcg./hour}} = 10.6 \text{ ml./hour}$

The client is on Hepathin anticoagulant therapy. The IV bag reads: Hepathin 30,000 units in 400ml of NS. Client weighs 140 pounds. Initial order: Hepathin 30,000 units in 400 ml of NS to infuse at 12 units per kilograms/hour. How many units are to be infused an hour for this person?_____ At what rate does the IV pump need to be set for this rate?____

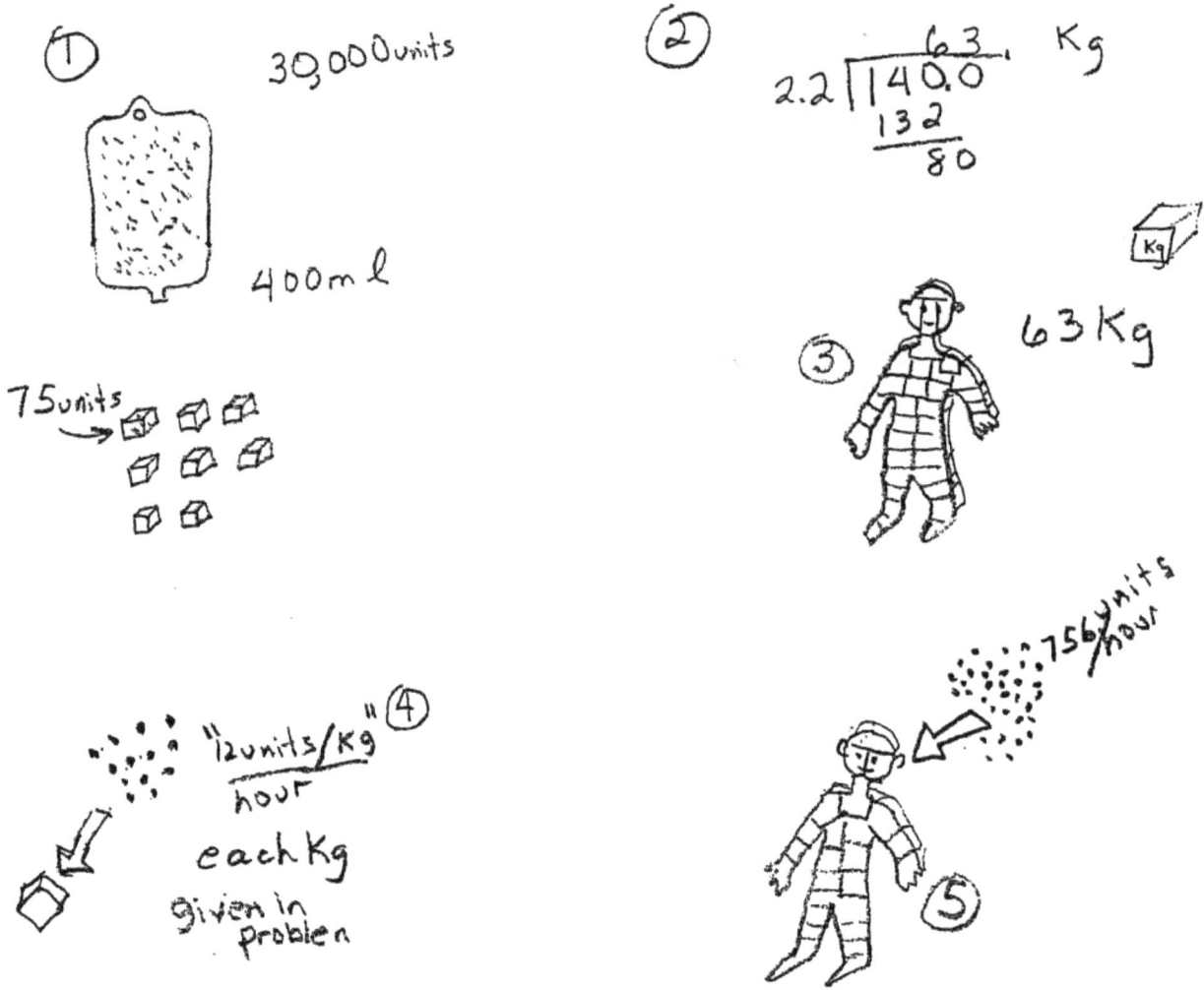

① 30,000 units

400 ml

75 units → ▢ ▢ ▢  ▢ ▢ ▢  ▢ ▢

② 
$$2.2\overline{)140.0} \quad Kg$$
$$\begin{array}{r} 63. \\ 132 \\ \hline 80 \end{array}$$

Kg

③ 63 Kg

④ "12 units/Kg"
hour
each Kg
given in problem

⑤ 756 units/hour

⑥ how many ml will it take to hold 756 units/hour

$$75\overline{)756} \quad \begin{array}{r} 10 \\ \end{array}$$ ml will hold 750
750

Set the pump @ 10ml/hour

First look at all of the extraneous and superfluous and useless information that is just meant to confuse you: *Mediex 600mg IV every six hours.* It doesn't matter what's in the juice or how often you have to do it. I never heard of Mediex.

The only thing that matters is 250 ml over 40 minutes. Intuitively that should sound fast.

$$\frac{250ml}{40\ min} = \frac{6.25ml}{min}$$

Each of those milliliters is 15 drops ( The drop factor is 15 gtt/ml).

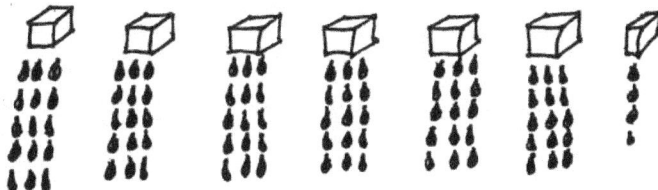

If 6.25 ml flow in one minute, how many drops will drip?

$$\frac{15gtts}{ml} \times \frac{6.25ml}{min} = \frac{93gtts}{min}$$

That's three drops every 2 seconds.

Now to set a pump: the pump is calibrated in ml/hour. You have to convert from ml/min to ml/hour.

If $\frac{6.25ml}{Min}$ must flow each minute then 60 times that amount must flow each hour. 375ml/hour. Like I said, that's fast.

One A.M. Medication Problem

The patient had a very labile blood pressure that could exceed 200 systolic or drop to 90. This probably was neurological but had to be controlled the old fashioned way with a nitro drip. As the evening progressed, so did the rate. When it reached 20 cc/hr I looked back at the original order. It said, "titrate nitro drip to keep sys b/p 130-140  Max 100 mics"

Say what? I looked at the bottle. It said, " 400 micrograms per cc." It also said, 100mg in a 250 cc bottle  You can see the label on page *102*

 "100 mics" must mean 100 micrograms per minute". How many cc's/hr would that be on the pump? I think the first thing to look at is how many mics would each cc/hr provide?

$$\frac{Hour}{60\ min} \times \frac{1cc}{hour} \times \frac{400mcg}{cc} = \frac{?mcg}{min}$$

$$\frac{1cc}{hour} = \frac{6.6mcg}{min}$$

That's "6.6 mics". I'm interested in 1 cc/hr because our pumps can only be raised or lowered 1cc/hr at a time.  If 1cc/hr is 6.67 mics, how many cc/hr will be 100mics?

$$\frac{?cc/hr}{1\ cc/hr} = \frac{100\ mics/min}{6.66\ mics/min}$$

15cc/hr would be 100 mics. The pump was going at 20cc/hr. Oops. Good idea to call the doctor. Turns out it wasn't too bad. He was in his car… awake. He said, "I guess the nitro isn't working. Let's try vasotec 2.5mg IV q4h prn for systolic greater than 140 and nitro at 100 mics. Then titrate nitro to keep systolic between 120 to 140."

The order is to give 200 ml of NS over one hour and then deliver the rest of the bag to 80 ml per hour. If the tubing has a drip factor of 12 gtts/ml, how many gtts/min will need to be counted per min to deliver the first dose?____How many gtts/min will need to be counted per min to deliver the second dose?_____ Thanks again for your help. Alesia

The next problem is not an unusual situation. In the case of dehydration, a lot of fluid quickly would be nice. Then a moderate flow maintains hydration.

200 ml over one hour is $\dfrac{200\ ml}{hour} = \dfrac{200\ ml}{60\ min} = \dfrac{3.33\ ml}{min}$

The picture shows that in 3.3 ml the are 39.96 gtt

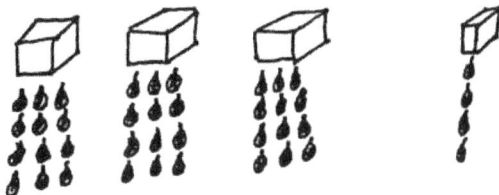

$\dfrac{3.3ml}{min} \times \dfrac{12\ gtt}{ml} = \dfrac{39.6\ gtt}{min}$

For the rest of the bag $\dfrac{80\ ml}{Hour} = \dfrac{1.3}{min}$

$\dfrac{1.3ml}{min} \times \dfrac{12\ gtt}{ml} = \dfrac{15.6gtt}{min}$

# QUICKLY CHECKING THE RATE

Do you remember in second grade how you checked subtraction problems? To check

$$\begin{array}{r} 7 \\ -3 \\ \hline 4 \end{array} \qquad \begin{array}{r} 4 \\ +3 \\ \hline 7 \end{array}$$

That is what we are doing here: working backwards from the answer to the question. You get report. You should get the order with the rate on the pump. You walk into the room, see the pump, see the concentration, and want to know if that is right for the order.

Lets look at vasopressin. We mix 200 units in 250 ml. D5W. The concentration is 0.8 ml./ml. The order is 0.2 units/min.

How many units is that an hour?

$$\frac{0.2\text{units}}{\text{min}} \times \frac{60\text{min}}{\text{hour}} = \frac{12 \text{ units}}{\text{hour}}$$

$$\frac{12 \text{ units/hour}}{0.8 \text{ units/ml}} = 15\text{ml/hr} \qquad \text{You would set the pump at 15ml/hr.}$$

Lets look at this calculation in pictures.

The order is 0.2 units/minute or 12 units/hour.

$$\frac{2}{10} u \Big\} \, min$$

∪ ∪ ∪ ∪ ∪ ∪
∪ ∪ ∪ ∪ ∪ ∪ } hour

How many ml./hr is that? (What do we set the pump at)

# Standard Drip Concentrations

| Drug | Class | Concentration | Solution | Dosage range | Rate |
|------|-------|---------------|----------|--------------|------|
| Abciximab | GPIIb/IIIa inhibitor | 9mg/250mL | Premixed/NS | Max 10mcg/min | mcg/kg/min |
| Aminocaproic acid | Hemostatic agent | 5gm/250mL | D$_5$W, NS | Max 30gm/day | gm/hr |
| Amiodarone | Antiarrhythmic | 450mg/250mL | D$_5$W | 1mg/min x 6hrs., 0.5mg/min x 18hrs. | mg/min |
| Amiodarone (bolus) | Antiarrhythmic | 150mg/100mL | D$_5$W | N/A | over 10 min. |
| Amrinone | Inotrope/Vasodilator | 100mg/100mL | NS | 5-10 mcg/kg/min | mcg/kg/min |
| Cisatracurium | Paralytic | 40mg/100mL | D$_5$W, NS | 0.5-10mcg/kg/min | mcg/kg/min |
| Dexmedetomidone | Sedative | 200mcg/50mL | NS | 0.2-0.7mcg/kg/hr | mcg/kg/hr |
| Diltiazem | Calcium channel blocker | 125mg/125mL | D$_5$W, NS | 2.5-15mg/hr | mg/hr |
| DoBUTamine | Inotrope | 500mg/250mL | Premixed/ D$_5$W | 2.5-20mcg/kg/min | mcg/kg/min |
| DOPamine | Catecholamine | 400mg/250mL | Premixed/ D$_5$W | 1-20mcg/kg/min | mcg/kg/min |
| Drotrecogin alfa | Activated protein C | 20mg/100mL | D$_5$W, NS | 24mcg/kg/hr x 96 hrs. | mcg/kg/hr |
| Epinephrine | Sympathomimetic | 8mg/250mL | D$_5$W, NS | 1-10mcg/min | mcg/min |
| Eptifibatide | GPIIb/IIIa inhibitor | 75mg/100mL | Premixed/SWFI | 2mcg/kg/min x 18-24 hrs. | mcg/kg/min |
| Esmolol | β-blocker | 2.5gm/250mL | Premixed/ D$_5$W | 50-300mcg/kg/min | mcg/kg/min |
| Fentanyl | Narcotic anagelsic | 1000mcg/100mL | D$_5$W, NS | 12.5-100mcg/hr | mcg/hr |
| Heparin | Anticoagulant | 25,000units/500mL | Premixed/ D$_5$W | Per protocol | units/hr |
| Insulin | Pancreatic hormone | 100units/100mL | NS | Per protocol | units/hr |
| Labetalol | β-blocker | 200mg/160mL | D$_5$W | 0.5-6mg/min | mg/min |
| Lidocaine | Antiarrhythmic | 2gm/500mL | Premixed/ D$_5$W | 1-4mg/min | mg/min |
| Lorazepam | Benzo. sedative | 50mg/50mL | NS | 1-4 mg/hr (titrate) | mg/hr |
| Midazolam | Benzo. sedative | 50mg/50mL | D$_5$W, NS | 0.5-5mg/hr (titrate) | mg/hr |
| Milrinone | Inotrope/Vasodilator | 20mg/10mL | D$_5$W, NS | 0.375-0.75mcg/kg/min | mcg/kg/min |
| Nesiritide | Natriuretic peptide | 1.5mg/250mL | D$_5$W, NS | 0.005-0.03mcg/kg/min | mcg/kg/min |
| Nitroglycerin | Vasodilator | 50mg/250mL | Premixed/ D$_5$W | 5-200mcg/min | mcg/min |
| Nitroprusside | Vasodilator | 50mg/250mL | D$_5$W | 0.5-10mcg/kg/min | mcg/kg/min |
| Norepinephrine | Sympathomimetic | 8mg/250mL | D$_5$W | 1-30mcg/min | mcg/min |
| Octreotide | Somatostatin analog | 500mcg/100mL | D$_5$W, NS | 25-100mcg/hr | mcg/hr |
| Phenylephrine | Sympathomimetic | 40mg/250mL | D$_5$W, NS | 5-200mcg/min | mcg/min |
| Procainamide | Antiarrhythmic | 2gm/500mL | D$_5$W, NS | 2-6mg/min | mg/min |
| Propofol | Sedative | 500mg/50mL | Premixed emulsion | 5-50mcg/kg/min | mcg/kg/min |
| Vecuronium | Paralytic | 50mg/250mL | D$_5$W, NS | 0.3-1.2mcg/kg/min | mcg/kg/min |

There are 0.8 units in each ml. (8 1/10ths).

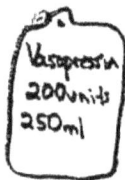

How many ml would we need to get 12 units/hr?

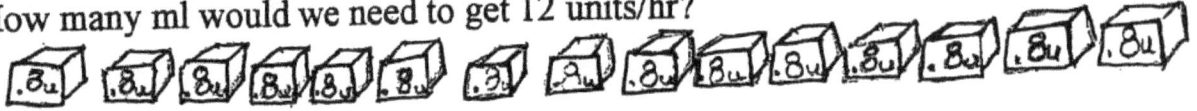

$$\frac{12\text{units/hour}}{0.8\text{ units/ml}} = 15\text{ml./hr}$$

# Now to check

That's how we got there. Lets go the other way. You walk into the room. The pump is set at 15cc/hour. The label says 200 units in 250 ml. That is 0.8 units in each ml. (8 1/10$^{th}$'s).

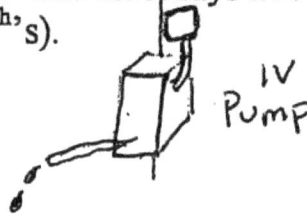

IV Bag

There are 0.8u/ml x 15 ml/hr = 12units/hr

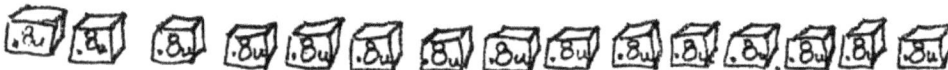

How many units are flowing each minute?

12 units divided by 60 is 0.2 units each minute

# IV DRIP "CHEAT SHEETS"

*Levophed/Norepinephrine Standard Conc.*
*8mg/250 ml D5W only*

*Vasopressin*
*160/250 = 0.44u/ml*
*0.24 = 30 ml/hr*
*0.34 = 46 ml/hr*
*0.44 = 60 ml/hr*

*25 u NS ... Vasopressin*

**EPINEPHRINE**
2 mg/250 NS = 8 mcg/ml
Dose: 1-4 mcg/min

1 mcg = 8 ml/hr
2 mcg = 15 ml/hr
3 mcg = 23 ml/hr
4 mcg = 30 ml/hr

**MAG SULFATE** –
preterm labor/PIH

Bolus dose: 4-6 gm/100 ml NS over 5-10 min.

Continuous 20 gm/500 ml NS
Infusion

1 gm/hr = 25 ml/hr
2 gm/hr = 50 ml/hr
3 gm/hr = 75 ml/hr
4 gm/hr = 100 ml/hr

Total Dose not to exceed 6 gm/hr.

ANTIDOTE: Ca Gluconate 10% (1 gm in 10 ml) IVP over 5 min.

**CARDIZEM**
Initial Dose: 0.25 mg/kg IVP over 2 min.
Usual Dose: 20 mg

Repeat Dose: (after 15 min.) 0.35 mg/kg IVP
Usual Dose: 30 mg.

Continuous 125 mg in 100 ml = 1 mg/ml
Infusion:
5 mg/hr = 5 ml/hr
10 mg/hr = 10 ml/hr
15 mg/hr = 15 ml/hr

**AMIODARONE**

For VF/VT: 300 mg in 20-30 ml D5W

For pulseless pts: 150 mg in 20-30 ml IVP over 10 min, followed by infusion.

Continuous infusion: 450 mg/250 ml D5W (Glass bottle) = 1.8 mg/ml
Infuse at 33 ml/hr X 6 hrs, then 17 ml/hr X 18 hrs.

**LIDOCAINE**
2 gm/250 ml = 8 mg/ml
Dose: 1-4 mg/min

1 mg = 8 ml/hr
2 mg = 15 ml/hr
3 mg = 23 ml/hr
4 mg = 30 ml/hr

**PITRESSIN**
200 units/250 ml = 0.8 u/ml
Dose: 0.2 - 0.4 u/min.
(Max: 0.9 u/min)

| per min | per hr |
|---|---|
| 0.2 units = 15 ml/hr |
| 0.3 units = 23 ml/hr |
| 0.4 units = 30 ml/hr |
| 0.5 units = 38 ml/hr |
| 0.6 units = 45 ml/hr |
| 0.7 units = 53 ml/hr |
| 0.8 units = 60 ml/hr |
| 0.9 units = 68 ml/hr |

**NITROGLYCERIN**
50 mg/250 ml D5W (Glass bottle) = 200 mcg/ml
3 ml = 10 mcg
Dose: Start 5 mcg/min and increase slowly.

5 mcg = 2 ml/hr
10 mcg = 3 ml/hr
20 mcg = 6 ml/hr
30 mcg = 9 ml/hr
40 mcg = 12 ml/hr
50 mcg = 15 ml/hr
60 mcg = 18 ml/hr
70 mcg = 21 ml/hr
80 mcg = 24 ml/hr
90 mcg = 27 ml/hr
100 mcg = 30 ml/hr

**NEO-SYNEPHRINE**
10 mg/250 ml D5W = 40 mcg/ml
Usual Dose: 10-60 mcg/min.

10 mcg = 15 ml
20 mcg = 30 ml
30 mcg = 45 ml
40 mcg = 60 ml
50 mcg = 75 ml
60 mcg = 90 ml

**DOBUTAMINE**
500 mg/250 ml D5W, NS = 2 mg/ml
Usual Dose: 2.5 – 20 mcg/kg/min

| Wt/lbs | 88 | 110 | 132 | 154 | 176 | 198 | 220 | 242 | 264 | 286 | 308 |
|---|---|---|---|---|---|---|---|---|---|---|---|
| Wt/kg | 40 | 50 | 60 | 70 | 80 | 90 | 100 | 110 | 120 | 130 | 140 |
| mcg/ 2.5 | 3 | 4 | 5 | 5 | 7 | 8 | 9 | 10 | 11 |
| kg/ 5 | 6 | 8 | 9 | 11 | 12 | 14 | 15 | 17 | 18 | 20 | 21 |
| min 10 | 12 | 15 | 18 | 21 | 24 | 27 | 30 | 33 | 36 | 39 | 42 |
| 15 | 18 | 23 | 27 | 32 | 36 | 41 | 45 | 50 | 54 | 59 | 63 |
| 20 | 24 | 30 | 36 | 42 | 48 | 54 | 60 | 66 | 72 | 78 | 84 |

Infusion Rate in ml/hr

**DOPAMINE**
800 mg/250 ml D5W or NS = 3.2 mg/ml
Dose: 2-20 mcg/kg/min.
Quick estimate: Take weight in lbs, drop last number, divide by two, set infusion pump to that number = approx. 5 mcg/kg/min.
Ex. 150 lbs = 5 mcg/kg/min at 7 ml/hr.

| Wt./lbs | | 88 | 110 | 132 | 154 | 176 | 198 | 220 | 242 | 264 | 286 | 308 |
| Wt. kg | | 40 | 50 | 60 | 70 | 80 | 90 | 100 | 110 | 120 | 130 | 140 |
|---|---|---|---|---|---|---|---|---|---|---|---|---|
| mcg/ | 2 | 2 | 2 | 2 | 3 | 3 | 3 | 4 | 4 | 5 | 5 | 5 |
| kg/ | 5 | 4 | 5 | 7 | 7 | 8 | 9 | 10 | 11 | 11 | 12 | 13 |
| min | 10 | 8 | 9 | 11 | 13 | 15 | 17 | 19 | 21 | 23 | 24 | 26 |
| | 15 | 11 | 14 | 17 | 20 | 23 | 25 | 28 | 31 | 34 | 37 | 40 |
| | 20 | 15 | 19 | 23 | 26 | 30 | 34 | 38 | 41 | 45 | 49 | 52 |

Infusion Rate in ml/hr

NOTE: For 400 mg/250 ml, double infusion rate

**DIPRIVAN**
1000 mg/100 ml = 10 mg/ml
Dose: 5-50 mcg/kg/min for sedation of VENTILATED pts.
Start at 5 mcg/kg and titrate 5-10 mcg every 5-10 min.

| Wt/lbs | | 88 | 110 | 132 | 154 | 176 | 198 | 220 | 242 | 264 | 286 | 308 |
| Wt/kg | | 40 | 50 | 60 | 70 | 80 | 90 | 100 | 110 | 120 | 130 | 140 |
|---|---|---|---|---|---|---|---|---|---|---|---|---|
| mcg/ | 5 | 1 | 2 | 2 | 2 | 2 | 3 | 3 | 3 | 4 | 4 | 4 |
| kg/ | 10 | 3 | 3 | 4 | 4 | 5 | 5 | 6 | 7 | 7 | 8 | 8 |
| min | 15 | 4 | 5 | 5 | 6 | 7 | 8 | 9 | 10 | 11 | 12 | 13 |
| | 20 | 5 | 6 | 7 | 8 | 10 | 11 | 12 | 13 | 14 | 16 | 17 |
| | 25 | 7 | 8 | 9 | 11 | 12 | 14 | 15 | 17 | 18 | 20 | 21 |
| | 30 | 8 | 9 | 11 | 13 | 14 | 16 | 18 | 20 | 22 | 23 | 25 |
| | 35 | 10 | 11 | 13 | 15 | 17 | 19 | 21 | 23 | 25 | 27 | 29 |
| | 40 | 11 | 12 | 14 | 17 | 19 | 22 | 24 | 26 | 29 | 31 | 33 |
| | 45 | 12 | 14 | 16 | 19 | 22 | 24 | 27 | 30 | 32 | 35 | 38 |
| | 50 | 14 | 15 | 18 | 21 | 24 | 27 | 30 | 33 | 36 | 39 | 42 |

Infusion Rate in ml/hr

**NIPRIDE**
50 mg/250 ml D5W only
Usual dose: 0.5 – 10 mcg/kg/min

| Wt/lb | | 88 | 110 | 132 | 154 | 176 | 198 | 220 | 242 | 264 | 286 | 308 |
| Wt/kg | | 40 | 50 | 60 | 70 | 80 | 90 | 100 | 110 | 120 | 130 | 140 |
|---|---|---|---|---|---|---|---|---|---|---|---|---|
| mcg/ | 0.5 | 12 | 14 | 14 | 15 | 17 | 18 | 20 | 21 |
| kg/ | 2 | 24 | 30 | 36 | 42 | 48 | 54 | 60 | 66 | 72 | 78 | 84 |
| min | 5 | 60 | 75 | 90 | 105 | 120 | 135 | 150 | 165 | 180 | 195 | 210 |
| | 7 | 84 | 105 | 126 | 147 | 168 | 189 | 210 | 231 | 252 | 273 | 294 |
| | 10 | 120 | 150 | 180 | 210 | 240 | 270 | 300 | 330 | 360 | 390 | 420 |

Infusion Rate in ml/hr

*Isuprel = 4mg/500u at 30cc/Hr = 4ug/min*

*7462*

# TRICKY MEDICATION PROBLEM

Here are some problems that were sent to me. They are interesting because they are tricky. I use that word because information is given in a way that distracts you from the medication calculation.

"A patient must receive grain 1/120 of scopolamine sc., a parasympathetic depressant. The label on the ampule reads 0.6 milligram per milliliter. How many minims will you administer to this patient?"

This is a trick problem. It would be like asking someone their car's gas mileage at a certain speed. Except, instead of miles per gallon at a certain miles per hour you used inches per pint of gas and yards per decade. Instead of how many miles per gallon does your car get at 65 miles per hour they asked, "How many inches per pint does your car get at 9,681,500,000 yards per decade?" I think that equals 65miles/hour. If it doesn't please let me know.

But the trick question was asked in a class and that makes it all the more relevant to this book. Whoever said life (and your medication test) wasn't tricky?

To answer the question I had to look up the definition of a minim. A minim is 1/16th ml or .06ml.

We know that a grain is 61mg. $1/120^{th}$ of a grain would be very close to 0.5mg. That's a reasonable amount. We need 0.5mg and there are 0.6mg/ml. Said a little differently, there are six $1/10^{th}$ mg. in each ml. But we only need five $1/10^{th}$ mg. How much fluid do we withdraw?

In an equation:
$$\frac{.5mg}{x} = \frac{0.6\ mg}{ml}$$

You would give 0.83ml. If a minim is 1/16 ml, that's 13.3 minims.

# TRICK PROBLEM #2

This one is more realistic but still tricky: The patient must receive 1,500,000 units of penicillin I.M. and the vial contains 20,000,000 units (in powdered form). The directions are as follows: add 38.7 ml sterile water to the vial. 1 ml = 500,000 units. How many milliliters will equal 1,500,000 units?

This is another trick problem. First there are units not milligrams you are used to and the numbers are very high (in the millions). Second you are inundated with information that confuses the question.

If you were given only the pertinent information, the question would be, "1 ml of penicillin = 500,000 units. How many ml will equal 1,500,000 units?" The answer, of course, is 3 ml.

All of the other facts are irrelevant and just meant to confuse you.

# MEDICAL JOKES

Cardiac Joke: What do you get when you spill a urinal?
Answer: see bottom of page

Immunology Joke: "I'm allergic to lasix. It makes me pee."

Hematology Joke: A vampire goes into a blood bank and asks for one unit of packed red cells and one unit of fresh frozen plasma. The phlebotomist yells back to the tech, "Gimme a Blud and a Blud Lite."

Otolaryngology Joke. For otitis media the doctor ordered "corticosporin drops in the R ear QID" The pharmacist called back to say corticosporin doesn't come in suppository form.

Orthopedic Joke (told by an infectious disease doctor): What do you need to do to pass the orthopedic boards? Be able to bench 200 pounds and spell Ancef.

Urology Joke: The doctor is doing a prostate exam. The guy yells, "That hurts!"
The doctor says," I'm using two fingers."
"Why?"
"I want a second opinion."

Infectious Disease Joke: How do you get a Kleenex to dance? Put a little boogie in it.

C.V. Joke: Did you hear about the two red blood cells who loved in vein?

To impress someone try saying, a gram of acetaminocin instead of two extra strength Tylenols.

G.I. Cartoon: There is a doctor, a nurse and a patient. The patient is draped and in the jack knife position presumabley for a sigmoidoscopy.. The nurse is holding a tray with a bottle of beer. The doctor with an angry look says, "No, I said I wanted a butt light."

I.C.U. Cartoon: There is a patient in an I.C.U. bed with monitors , dynamaps, oxygen, and all the familiar paraphanalia. He is talking on the phone saying, "Bells are ringing and the T.V.has a straight line."

A guy goes in to see a doctor. He touches his head and says, every time I touch it here it hurts." He touches his stomach and says the same thing. He touches his knee and repeats it again. The doctor examines him and says, "Your finger is broken."

Answer to cardiology joke: You get a Pee Wave

A very attractive young man and a vivacious young lady meet in a fashionable night club and they hit it off immediately. Later in the evening they discuss spending the night together and leave immediately for the woman's apartment. As they are getting ready for bed the woman goes into the bathroom and starts to compulsively wash her hands for an excessive length of time. The man asks, "Are you a doctor?"

"Yes."

"Don't tell me! A surgeon! Right?"

"Yes. How did you know?"

"It was obvious. I could see your concern for transmitting germs and preventing infection."

They go have sex and afterward, the woman asks the man, "Are you a doctor?"

"Yes."

"Don't tell me! An anesthesiologist! Right?"

"Yes. How did you know?"

"I didn't feel a thing."


Ophthalmology Joke: This takes place in a very exclusive private girls' school. The eighth grade science teacher, Mr. Johnson, asks, " What organ of the body, when stimulated, expands to six times its normal size? Miss Smith?"

"Mr. Johnson, I don't think that is a proper question to ask a girl of my age and social standing."

He calls on another student, "Miss Jones?"

"The pupil of the eye"

"That is correct. Miss Smith I have three things to say to you. One: you didn't do your homework. Two: you have a dirty mind. Three: someday you are going to be very disappointed."


Orthopedic Joke. A guy sees a doctor. He says, "Everywhere I touch it hurts." He touches his forehead and says, "It hurts." He touches his stomach and says the same thing. He touches his knee. Again, same thing. The doctor says, "Let me examine you." After a few minutes of poking and prodding, "Your finger is broken."


Ask any surgeon to name the three best surgeons in the world. They'll have a hard time thinking of the other two.


"Do you know the definition of "innuendo"?

"Yeah sure. That's simple"

explanatory of the text
²innuendo *also* inuendo \˙\ *n, pl* innuendos *or* innuendoes 1 : veiled, oblique, or covert allusion to something not directly named : HINT, INSINUATION (glossy fantasy, stylishness, naughty ~ —*Time*) (a talk punctuated with ~s on both sides —J.T.Farrell); *esp* : veiled or equivocal allusion reflecting upon the character, ability, or other trait of the person referred to (try to undermine him by ~ —*Kiplinger Washington Letter*) (how difficult it is to set up a proper defense against ~ —M.S.Watson) (anonymous accusations, rumors, ~s —Nathan Schachner) 2 : a parenthetical explanation of the text of a legal document; *esp* : an interpretation in a pleading of expressions alleged to be injurious or libelous
³innuendo *also* inuendo \˙\ *vb* -ED/-ING/-S [¹innuendo] *vi*

"No. It's an Italian enema."

Plastic Surgery: During routine surgery a woman goes into cardiac arrest. After superhuman efforts and being apparently dead she miraculously recovers. During this ordeal she has an out-of-body experience in which she talks to God. God tells her she get forty more years to live and she should make the most of it be striving to be her best. From that she concludes she should improve her appearance and has liposuction, breast augmentation and a face lift. As she is leaving the hospital a bus hits her and instantly kills her. When she gets to heaven she asks God," What's this all about? You said..." God interrupts, "I didn't recognize you."

Surgery: How does a surgeon change a light bulb? They Just hold it in the socket and stand still. The earth revolves around them.

Psychiatry: How many psychiatrists does it take to change a light bulb?
Only one. But first, the light bulb has to want to change.

A man on a crowded bus a man sees a woman with grocery bags and two small children. He gets up to give her his seat and helps her with the bags.
"Thank you. You're sweet" she says.
"I know. I'm diabetic."
Thanks to Dr. Murray Miller, an endocrinologist, for that one.

How do you tell the difference between an oral thermometer and a rectal thermometer? The taste.

Q: Why are barracuda and sharks so healthy?
A: They eat fish.

Q: What is the cause of inverted P-waves?
A: Hypospadia

Q: What is the therapeutic effect of mixing Rogaine and Viagra?
A: Don King

A busy urologist's office answers the phone, "Urology Associates. Can you hold?"

Q: What did the epididymis say to the seminal vesicle?
A: "There is a vas deferens between us"

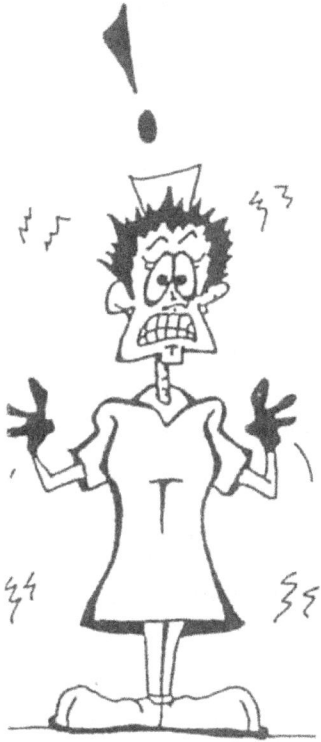
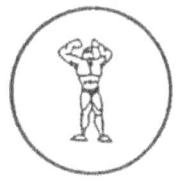
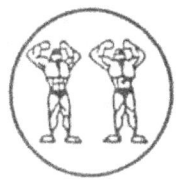
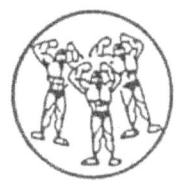
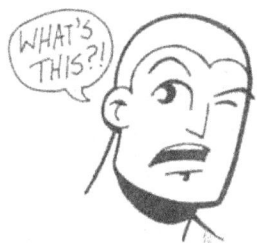

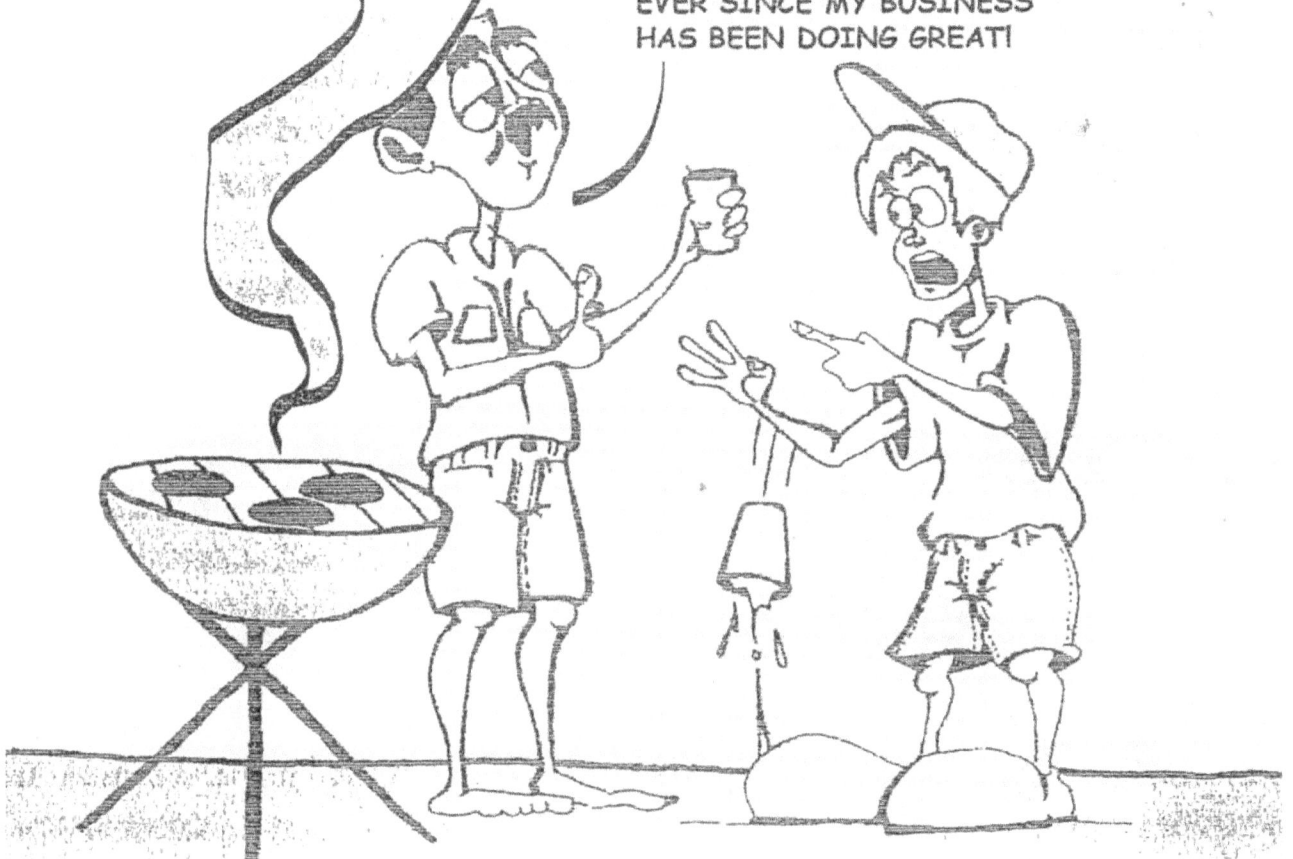

Drug Calculations For Nurses Who Hate Numbers ©1992

Retail: $18.95

ISBN 0-9725483-0-0

9780972548304

0 700814 497989

7 00814 49798 9

www.ingramcontent.com/pod-product-compliance
Lightning Source LLC
Chambersburg PA
CBHW062027210326

41519CB00060B/7192